PREVENTING PATIENT FALLS

To *Nora Morrow*, B.Sc.N., R.N.
For her belief in research and her faith in people

And for my father
Percy Joseph Hambleton
who once fell 1,000 feet

PREVENTING PATIENT FALLS

JANICE M. MORSE

SAGE Publications
International Educational and Professional Publisher
Thousand Oaks   London   New Delhi

For information address:

 SAGE Publications, Inc.
2455 Teller Road
Thousand Oaks, California 91320
E-mail: order@sagepub.com

SAGE Publications Ltd.
6 Bonhill Street
London EC2A 4PU
United Kingdom

SAGE Publications India Pvt. Ltd.
M-32 Market
Greater Kailash I
New Delhi 110 048 India

Printed in the United States of America

Library of Congress Cataloging-in-Publication Data

Morse, Janice M.
    Preventing patient falls / author, Janice M. Morse.
       p.   cm.
    Includes bibliographical references and index.
    ISBN 0-7619-0592-8 (cloth). — ISBN 0-7619-0593-6 (pbk.)
    1. Health facilities—Safety measures.   2. Falls (Accidents)—
Prevention.   I. Title.
RA969.9.M67   1996
362.1′068′4—dc20   96-10145

97 98 99 00 01 02 03 10 9 8 7 6 5 4 3 2 1

Acquiring Editors:	Dan Ruth and Harry Briggs
Editorial Assistants:	Nancy Hale and Jessica Crawford
Production Editor:	Vicki Baker
Production Assistant:	Sherrise Purdum
Typesetter/Designer:	Janelle LeMaster
Art Director:	Ravi Balasuriya

a 703 236

WA 250

Contents

Appendixes

Preface

Read Me

This book has arisen out of research conducted between 1983 and 1989 examining patient falls, research on patient restraints (1985-1988), projects to develop a safe hospital bed and bed alarm (1986-1991), and the implementation of fall prevention programs at many institutions in Canada and the United States. Most important, the book is a result of hundreds of questions asked by clinicians as they have struggled to apply the research to practice—to use the research by implementing a fall prevention program. This book is dedicated to those concerned clinical nurse specialists who clearly go the extra mile to provide excellent patient care.

Nursing, at the present time, is in a difficult period. There has been much discussion about whose responsibility it is to make research applicable to practice, to prepare it in a form that can be used prescriptively. As a researcher, I have actively resisted being forced into taking this step: I have enough to do doing research and have argued that if I take time out to rewrite my work, this will impede current research. Besides, I argued arrogantly, my writing is clear.

Perhaps my writing is clear to *me*, but it was less clear to clinicians because questions kept coming. Often, these questions appeared far removed from anything I had imagined or expected. For example, I was asked: "How do you score an unconscious patient [for fall risk]?" "Under what circumstances," I asked, "can an unconscious patient fall?" "Well," I was told, "if a nurse turning a patient in bed forgot to put the side rail up and the patient rolled onto the floor." That, to me, appears to be a *drop*—not a fall—and a dropped patient hasn't fallen. I became frustrated because administrators wanted to know—and for me to tell them—exactly when a patient should be scored with the *Morse Fall Scale* and what score was high risk. I considered these decisions to be the prerogative of the administrator and to involve many other factors that I had no control over, such as how much risk administrators were willing to assume and what resources administrators were willing to provide to assist with the prevention of falls. It is a risk:benefit ratio: The acceptable fall rate may be determined by the number chosen as risk level on the Fall Scale. If administration decides that their institution will have a low fall rate (and is willing to provide the environmental and staff resources to pay for the low fall rate), then the Scale is set as low as reasonably possible. Obviously, setting the Scale too low—so that most of the patients on the unit are considered high risk—is more costly than considering only a third of the patients to be high risk. Therefore, although I can make recommendations based on experience using the Scale, the setting of the scale is an administrator's decision. But most important, the areas of misunderstanding made it clear that research articles describing the development of the Scale were inadequate for implementation of fall prevention programs in the clinical setting.

A second insight came when administrators and nursing staff wanted me to make clear recommendations for interventions and often wanted me to make recommendations that extended directly from the patient's score. It become evident that staff did not know what to expect from the Morse Fall Scale. The Morse Fall Scale is a predictor of the likelihood of falling, not a diagnostic tool. Think of it as a thermometer: A thermometer tells the nurse only when an infection is present, but it gives no information as to where the infection is or which antibiotic to use. Similarly, the Morse Fall Scale will tell you who is likely to fall and will even give an indication of the probability that the patient will fall. But the Scale will not diagnose the problem or recommend preventive strategies. The Scale gives no information about when or where the patient will fall nor how to prevent the fall. The diagnosis and the identification of fall prevention strategies are patient specific, and the task of the expert nurse-clinician and his or her consultants is to identify strategies to prevent the fall and to develop an appropriate prevention plan. A book was needed to clear this confusion.

The third reason for writing this book was that I indirectly heard of "disasters," or approaches to fall prevention, that were enough to give me nightmares. For example, I heard of the Morse Fall Scale being used routinely in a clinical setting to identify the fall-prone patient without a well-developed and coordinated plan for preventing falls. There is more to a fall-prevention program than using a fall scale. A fall prevention program consists of five interrelated components described in Chapter 1 and detailed throughout this book. Using the Scale alone, without the coordinated supporting components, places the institution and staff in jeopardy. I could imagine a serious injury resulting from a fall, a subsequent lawsuit, and a lawyer asking the staff: "You knew this patient's fall risk score was 85, at high risk of falling, yet you made no attempt to prevent the fall?" The lack of a book—a manual—resulted in too many misunderstandings and expectations about the Scale, its limitations, and its purpose.

Fourth, and related to the previous point—the Scale was given, I felt, undue credit. Nurses who used the Morse Fall Scale reported, for example, that "Falls were reduced by 50% percent." The Scale itself does not *prevent* falls; rather, the nurses' preventive strategies targeted at fall-prone patients make the difference. The Scale merely informs the staff about where to place their energies or on which patients to focus their attention. It takes some of the guess work out of fall prevention.

Finally, I heard the frustration of nurses at the bedside using the Morse Fall Scale and identifying the patients at risk of falling; when they received no support from administration for extra staff, they used restraints to prevent the predicted fall. It was apparent that the nurses and administration had to realize that fall prevention was not something that could be set as an institutional objective without administration accepting responsibility for the concomitant costs for additional staffing or environmental supports. I had to make this risk clear.

Therefore, in light of the increasing weight from the above five reasons to write, I have reluctantly produced this book. I hope that by reorganizing the set of publications into a more intelligible whole, these five problems will fade away.

Doing this research has been an interesting process. When that Scale was first developed with Suzanne Tylko and Robert Morse, it was clear that it was really "spot on" for predicting patient falls, but I didn't know how to prevent those falls. I knew that by releasing the Scale, nurses would feel in a bind knowing who was likely to fall, but not knowing what to do about it. I feared that nurses, not knowing how to prevent a fall, would increase restraint use. Thus, I delayed the publication of the Scale until I studied restraints and the efficacy of bed alarms. I realized that full-length side rails were lethal, lobbied to have them removed, and lost. I developed specifications for a safe low-high bed, and this was patented, but because of the lack of a business partner, it has not been manufactured. With Julian Stedman, I developed a cheap and reliable bed alarm and spent several years testing the prototype in clinical areas, but, again, this is not yet available commercially.

Therefore, this manual for clinicians is the final step in my research program for preventing patient falls. As explained, the manual was written first for administrators. The bottom line is that I do not recommend that a fall prevention program be instituted without institutional commitment, because nurses at the bedside cannot prevent falls without your support and without resources. Institutional commitment means dollars—not too many—but enough to provide adequate staffing, safe equipment, and equipment that is in good repair. It may mean modifying a unit, replacing dangerous equipment, or installing hand rails. It means negotiating (i.e., instructing/ordering) with other hospital departments on behalf of nurses for minor changes in procedures that will assist in increasing patient safety. It means administrating responsibly.

Researchers cannot solve all the problems: It is ironic that for 5 years, I was unsuccessful in persuading the housekeeping department to replace the shiny floor polish and to use a matte, nonslip, and nonglare sealer. I argued that the shiny surface caused falls by interfering with the vision of the elderly resident. Despite documentation of the hazards, the value of "cleanliness" as evidenced by a shiny floor had greater priority than patient comfort and safety. Only the upper echelons of administration have the power to decree such changes—not the nurses, not the patients, and certainly not the researcher!

Next, this book is written for the nurse at the bedside providing patient care. The burden of preventing falls has been placed firmly on your shoulders. Your wisdom and judgment, your observational skills, and your past experiences provide an excellent background for you to develop a repertoire of innovative and creative ways to prevent patients from falling. The irony of your position is evident—if you do prevent the fall, there is little or no acknowledgment of your success, for if a fall is successfully prevented, as a statistic, it hasn't happened! But if a patient falls—and some do—the burden of the incident may be placed on your shoulders. Insist that administrators support you in your endeavor, for you cannot prevent falls without their help, their funding, and their encouragement.

Finally, the book is written for other researchers. Although I am clearly presenting my own research program, if there are other instruments or forms that may be used, I will review those alternatives. Data needed for the assessment of the reliability and validity of the Morse Fall Scale or to establish a fall prevention program have been placed in appendixes.

Patient falls are extremely complex phenomena to study, with diverse causality and an infinite variety of prevention strategies. Furthermore, although contributing factors such as gait and balance have been explored under controlled conditions, it is not possible to experimentally stage a patient fall, and therefore, research is confined to the "naturalistic setting" of the institution. One cannot study predictors of the fall without ethically and morally simultaneously taking steps to prevent the fall. Thus, the researcher finds him- or herself in the extraordinary position of implementing a program that both predicts and prevents the outcome variable (i.e., the fall). Thus, if a prevention program is successful, theoretically, there should be no data! I overcame this difficulty somewhat in the prospective study of falls (reported in Appendix E), by collecting data on "missed falls"; that is, falls that had almost occurred but somehow were prevented. For example, if a nurse was called to the room by the sounding of the bed alarm and found the patient in a precarious position, climbing out of bed, or if a patient was caught as he or she collapsed, and a fall was prevented, I collected these incidents as data. This is rather peculiar evidence for "success," but it was the best research design that could be developed.

Research is not conducted alone. I am indebted for the assistance and support of the following people. Research assistants and collaborators were Nora Morrow, Gail Federspeil, Suzanne Tylko, Herb Dixon, Pat Donahue, Ruth Tuck, Gail O'Connor, Colleen Black, and Kathy Oberle. Sharon Warren, Steve Hunka, and Robert Morse have assisted with data analysis. Randy Roberson and Dennis Bowers assisted with the preparation of a video. Pat Donahue, Julian Stedman, and Dean Olmstead were involved with the development of the hospital bed and the bed alarm. Caroline Rudd, Janice Penrod, and Gail Havens, supported this effort by reading the manuscript, and Susan Dolan and Anna Lombard provided editorial assistance. More than 400 nurses in two institutions were involved with the prospective component of testing the Scale. And many residents and patients have been interviewed, examined, and obligingly climbed in and out of bed or walked for us while we observed their gait.

The copyright for the Morse Fall Scale is held by the *Canadian Journal on Aging,* and I thank them for their permission to reproduce it here. For internal institutional use, the Scale may be duplicated as needed, provided three conditions are met: (a) the items must not be changed—that is, do not omit an item or change the score value of any item; (b) please advise me of the results obtained from the use of the Scale and of any problem that you have with its use—in this way, the Scale can, if necessary, be modified; and (c) if the Scale is published with results of your implementation, appropriate copyright permission must be obtained from the *Canadian Journal on Aging.*

I am grateful for the permission to reprint previously published material from

> *Canadian Journal of Public Health*
> *The Gerontologist*
> *Canadian Journal on Aging*
> *Social Science & Medicine*
> *QRB: Quality Review Bulletin*
> *Journal of Gerontological Nursing*
> *Annual Review of Nursing Research*
> *Research in Nursing and Health*

Financial support was provided for this research by the Alberta Foundation for Nursing Research, Alberta Association of Registered Nurses, University of Alberta Hospitals, University of Alberta Hospitals Foundation, University of Alberta Central Research Fund, Alberta Medical Heritage Research Fund, and through a NHRDP Research Scholar Award. And last, but not least, I am grateful to Christine Smedley, Senior Nursing Editor at Sage Publications, for her gentle reminders to complete the "Falls Project," and to Harry Briggs for seeing it through.

Janice M. Morse
February 1996

1

Creating a Fall Prevention Program

An Overview

Once considered an "accident" and an unavoidable problem of illness, disability, or advancing age, falls were accepted as a normal consequence of being ill, and any injury resulting from the fall was accepted as "bad luck." However, research on falls has escalated in the past 15 years, and presently, falls are considered an event that may be predicted with reasonable certainty and therefore prevented. In the past 5 years, caregivers and patient advocacy groups have become vocal about care of the elderly, and restraining the confused elderly patient[1] to prevent a fall is no longer acceptable. Technical developments have improved, so that when a patient attempts to get out of bed unassisted or to leave the unit, alarms sound to alert the caregiver.

Despite these advances, many things remain unchanged. Bed design has not changed dramatically, although it has been documented extensively that most patient falls occur when the patient is attempting to get out of bed without assistance. The design of wheelchairs has not been dramatically altered, and transfer boards are still needed for some patients when moving from the wheelchair to the bed. And despite research into the prediction of falls, some research is still published reporting fall rates from retrospective chart reviews from one institution or another. Clearly, it is time that fall rates were accepted as standard and used only to assist clinicians to evaluate a fall prevention program.

Standardized fall rates assist clinicians to evaluate a fall prevention program and to compare fall rates with other institutions.

The main purpose of this book is to present almost a decade of research into patient falls that constitute a research program and to present the research in a form that is useful to hospital administrators and nurses. The primary objective is to provide instruction on how to develop a program using the Morse Fall Scale.

Despite the recent advances into understanding patient falls, falls remain a major problem. Falls have been identified as the second leading cause of accidental death in the United States, and 75% of those falls occur in the elderly population. When hospitalized, patients are placed in jeopardy. They are weakened from the illness, from surgery, and from bed rest; they may feel unwell and unsteady as a result of receiving multiple medications; they may experience conditions that force them to rush to the bathroom, such as urinary frequency or urgency or diarrhea; they are placed in a strange environment where the furniture is arranged differently and is disconcertingly disproportionate; and they must rely on asking strangers for assistance with intimate bodily functions.

Of primary importance is that when a patient falls in the hospital, 6% of those falls result in serious injuries that further compromise health status or even result in death, either from the fall or secondary causes. Injuries from falls dramatically increase health care costs, estimated at billions of dollars annually (Baker & Harvey, 1985).

> When a patient falls, 6% of those falls result in serious injuries that further compromise health status or even result in death.

The Problem of Patient Falls

What is a fall? One of the problems in conducting fall research is defining the fall itself. Morris and Isaacs (1980) define a fall as "an untoward event in which the patient comes to rest unintentionally on the floor" (p. 181). But this definition is problematic for clinicians. Has the patient fallen if the patient is "caught" and lowered into a chair? Is it considered a fall if the patient grabs a handrail and does not fall on the floor? And is it considered a fall if a nurse finds a patient on the floor, but the patient cannot tell the nurse what happened and the event was not witnessed? My only advice is to use your best judgment. And it seems to me that all of the scenarios described above may be considered a fall and reported as such.

It is incredibly important to *report all falls*. The reason is that once the patient has fallen, he or she is particularly likely to fall a second time. Furthermore, the odds suggest that the patient will fall a second time doing the same thing. Thus, although the most important aspect of prevention is to predict the fall before it occurs, it is also important to examine and record the circum-

> Examine and record the circumstances surrounding the fall so that a reoccurrence may be prevented.

stances surrounding the fall so that recurrence may be prevented.

Falls occur in all types of health care institutions and to all patient populations. Table 1.1 shows fall rates for some types of patient populations. Notice that the rates are lowest in the general, acute care

Table 1.1 Comparison of Patient Fall Rates[a] for Various Patient Populations

Author	Fall Rate	Patient Population	Comments
General hospital			
Cohen and Guin (1991)	3.8	Adult neuroscience	1-year period
Kilpack, Boehm, Smith, and Mudge (1991)	4.7 4.1 3.0-3.6	Medical-surgical unit Medical-surgical unit Total hospital	
Llewellyn, Martin, Shekleton, and Firlit (1988)	3.8	Cardiovascular surgical unit	3.4-4.4/mth. yr. 1
Morgan, Mathison, Rice, and Clemmer (1985)	3.35	Acute care hospital	
Morse, Black, Oberle, and Donahue (1989)	2.5	1,200-bed general hospital (including 140-bed nursing home + 50-bed geriatric center)	Average over 10-year period
Raz and Baretich (1987)	2.18 2.53	University hospital VA hospital	
Rehabilitation hospital			
Mion et al. (1989)	46/143 patients fell	Of 46 patients, 29 fell more than once	
Vlahov, Myers, and Al-Ibrahim (1990)	178 falls per 1000 *patients* per year		
Nursing home/long-term care			
Berry, Fisher, and Lang (1981)	4.27	50.9% of patients fell more than once, accounting for 79.53% of all falls	
Morris and Isaacs (1980)	422 falls per 1,000 patients at risk		
Myers et al. (1989)	5.7		

a. Unless otherwise stated, patient fall rate = (# falls/# patient bed days) × 1,000 hospitals and highest in the nursing homes, with the rates in the rehabilitation hospitals falling somewhere in between. These rates are important because they give the clinician

> When a fall prevention program is first initiated, fall rates *escalate* because of increased reporting.

some basis for comparison as the rates in one's own institution are recorded and better understood. However, in reality, a fall is a fairly uncommon event. This means that the statistics can be inflated easily if a fall rate is estimated for a small group (such as a unit) for a short period of time. In this case, several falls (or one patient falling repeatedly) could inflate the fall rate, and we see this phenomenon in some of the statistics on Table 1.1 (see Kilpack, Boehm, Smith, & Mudge, 1991). When the patient population is increased (as with reporting on the entire hospital, especially over the period of a year or more), then the fall rate becomes more stable. Another important point is that when a program is first initiated, fall rates *escalate* because of the enthusiastic reporting by staff members. For this reason, it is also important to record *injury rates.* Although an injury is a less frequent occurrence, a fall that results in an injury is always reported. The injury rates tend to be more reliable, and therefore more stable, than do fall rates. This aspect of recording will be discussed later.

Identifying Types of Falls

Patients fall for a large variety of reasons, and if falls are to be prevented, it is critical to understand the etiology of a fall.[2] Analysis of circumstances surrounding 100 patients who fell and 100 randomly selected patients who had not fallen (Morse, Tylko, & Dixon, 1987) revealed that three types of patient falls occurred in hos-

> Identifying falls as *anticipated physiological falls, unanticipated physiological falls,* or *accidental falls* is important because methods for prediction and prevention differ for each type of fall.

pitals and long-term care institutions. Because there are different causes of falls, the strategies for preventing patient falls are different for each type of fall. A fall may be classified as *accidental* or *physiological*. The physiological falls are further classified as predictable—that is, an *anticipated physiological fall* (i.e., the patient exhibits signs that indicate the likelihood of falling and scores at-risk on the Morse Fall Scale)—or as unpredictable—that is, an *unanticipated physiological fall*.

    1. *Accidental falls.* Fourteen percent of all falls are considered accidental, caused by the patient slipping, tripping, or having some other mishap that results in a fall. These falls are often caused by environmental factors such as spilled water or urine on the floor. A patient may fall when using an IV stand for support when the wheels stick suddenly or he or she may fall when the top of the IV pole catches on an overhead curtain railing or doorway. Alternatively, the patient may fall when climbing out of bed if the bed is in an unexpectedly high position. Accidental falls also may be caused by the patient making errors of judgment, such as leaning against a curtain, thinking it was a supportive wall; misjudging the width of a doorway and not realizing that the doorways in institutions are wider than those in the home; or leaning on a bedside locker and having the locker suddenly roll away. Accidental falls also may occur when the patient loses balance while ambulating. For instance, the patient may be rising from a chair and reaching for a walker, leaning from the bed and reaching for an object, using poor technique when transferring, or forgetting to lift the foot pedal of the wheelchair before standing. It is important to note that the patient who experiences an accidental fall may not have been identified as being at risk of falling on the Morse Fall Scale.

    Because accidental falls are not due to physical factors but rather environmental hazards or errors of judgment, prevention strategies

> Fourteen percent of all falls are considered *accidental,* caused by the patient slipping, tripping, or having some other mishap that results in a fall.

are designed to ensure that the environment is free from hazards, that the patient is oriented to the environment and has received instruction on how to use walkers, and so forth. This includes instruction on the correct method of transferring from a wheelchair.

> *Anticipated physiological falls* (78% of falls) occur when residents who score "at risk of falling" on the Morse Fall Scale subsequently fall.

2. *Anticipated physiological falls.* These are falls that occur with the patients identified as fall-prone by scoring "at risk of falling" on the Morse Fall Scale. The items on the Morse Fall Scale are based upon research findings and represent six factors that contribute significantly to the patient's likelihood of falling (Morse, Morse, & Tylko, 1989). These factors are the following: more than one diagnosis, a previous fall, a weak or impaired gait, the lack of a realistic assessment of his or her own abilities to go to the bathroom unassisted, an IV or heparin lock, and an ambulatory aid. Anticipated physiological falls constitute 78% of all falls.

3. *Unanticipated physiological falls.* These are falls that may be attributed to physiological causes but are created by conditions that *cannot be predicted* before the first occurrence. They constitute approximately 8% of all falls. Examples of physiological conditions that result in unanticipated physiological falls include seizures, "drop attacks," fainting, or a pathological fracture of the hip. When this type

> *Unanticipated physiological falls* may be attributed to physiological causes that *cannot be predicted* before the first fall.

of fall occurs and there is a likelihood that the underlying condition may recur, nursing attention is targeted toward either preventing a second fall or preventing injury when the patient falls again. For example, nurses may teach a patient with orthostatic hypotension how to recognize the dizziness on rising and how to get up slowly, thus reducing the risk of falling.

To emphasize, differentiating falls into anticipated and unanticipated physiological falls and accidental falls is important because
methods for prediction and
prevention differ for each type
of fall. The Morse Fall Scale
predicts anticipated physiological falls; prevention strategies
are to develop an individualized fall prevention program
that will lower the patient's risk
score and prevent the fall. Accidental falls cannot be predicted using
the scale. They are prevented by making the environment as safe as
possible. Unanticipated physiological falls cannot be predicted using
the scale nor prevented from occurring the first time. Prevention is
targeted toward strategies for protecting the patient from a second
fall. The notion of protection is important because sometimes the fall
cannot be prevented. Rather, protection strategies are taken to ensure
that the patient does not injure him- or herself in the fall. For example,
a patient with epilepsy may fall in the process of having a seizure, and
this cannot be predicted or changed. But the protective strategy would
be to teach that patient how to protect his or her head or to ensure
that the patient wears a helmet to prevent head injury should a seizure
occur. Many patients, such as those with Parkinson's disease, can be
taught how to fall.

*The Morse Fall Scale predicts physi-
ological anticipated falls.*

Collecting Baseline Data

The first step, before making the decision to initiate a fall prevention program, is to ascertain whether or not patient falls are a problem
in the institution and, if falling is a problem, to gain an estimate of
how serious the problem is. The fastest way to evaluate the problem
is to analyze the institution's incident report forms used for reporting
a fall. Tabulate all falls and all injuries that have resulted from a fall,
preferably for a 12-month period. Calculate the fall rate and the injury

rate for the institution using the formula for *fall rates* and *injury rates* presented in Appendix D. If incident report forms are not available for analysis, then it will be necessary to collect fall statistics for a predetermined length of time, preferably for at least 3 months. *Warning:* Reviewing fall statistics, causes of falls, and the literature, it is tempting to ignore or "improve" on the literature by creating your own fall scale by selecting items from several scales, or even by writing your own items. Such efforts probably will have no reliability or validity, and they will not be predictive of falling. Save your time and energy, and select a scale that has reported reliability and validity and meets the needs of your institution. Altering scale items, or altering scale scores, will destroy a scale's reliability and validity. Scales are not created arbitrarily and should not be altered.

Planning a Fall Prevention Program

Because there are three types of patient falls (i.e., the accidental fall, the anticipated physiological fall, and the unanticipated physiological fall), approaches and methods of fall prevention differ with each type of fall. The comprehensive fall prevention program is therefore sorted into three components, each targeted to prevent a fall or to protect the patient who is likely to fall.

> The comprehensive fall prevention program is therefore sorted into three components, each targeted to prevent a fall or to protect the patient who is likely to fall.

The first type of fall, the *accidental fall*, is prevented by ensuring a safe environment so that an accidental fall will not occur. Whereas accidental falls are likely to occur in patients with a normal gait, they are more likely to occur in patients who have an abnormal gait. For instance, pa-

> The *accidental fall* is prevented by ensuring a safe environment.

tients with an impaired gait who shuffle and cannot lift their feet are more likely to trip. Accidental falls are prevented by ensuring a safe environment, and the process and procedures for checking the environment are described in Chapter 2.

Anticipated physiological falls are prevented by first identifying who is likely to fall by administering the Morse Fall Scale. Those patients who score at high or medium risk of falling are then assessed to see if the possible cause of the fall may be corrected or reduced (e.g., by altering medications to reduce confusion, using physiotherapy to increase muscle strength and improve gait, or providing correct instruction for the use of a walker, etc.). Another approach may be to identify a nursing care plan to reduce fall risk, such as waking the patient at night for toileting, or else increasing surveillance. Alternatively, special equipment, such as bean bag chairs or bed alarms, can be used to ensure safety or assist with patient monitoring.

> *Anticipated physiological falls* are prevented by first identifying who is likely to fall using the Morse Fall Scale.

The first unanticipated physiological fall cannot be prevented because the staff and the patient may not realize that the patient has the condition that suddenly precipitates the fall (i.e., a seizure). In this case, the approach is to *protect the patient* by preventing injury should a second fall occur (e.g., by requiring the patient to wear a helmet to protect head injury or by teaching the patient with orthostatic hypotension to rise from a chair slowly). Each of these approaches is highlighted in Figure 1.1 with references made to the sections that detail each approach.

> The first *unanticipated patient fall* cannot be prevented—protect the patient by preventing injury should a second fall occur.

Multidimensional Approaches to Fall Prevention

- Prevent *Accidental Falls* by
  1. Ensuring a safe environment (Chapter 2)

- Prevent *Anticipated Physiological Falls* by
  1. Identifying the fall-prone patients using the Morse Fall Scale (Chapter 4)
  2. Conducting a fall assessment on each patient determined at risk of falling (Chapter 4)
  3. Identifying fall prevention strategies for each patient at risk of falling (Chapter 5)

- Prevent injury from the recurrence of *Unanticipated Physiological Falls* by
  1. Protecting patients should they fall again (Chapter 5)

- Establish a procedure of continuous monitoring of falls (Chapter 6)

Figure 1.1. Overview of Fall Prevention Program

Institutional Coordination for Fall Prevention

Preventing patient falls requires a planned and coordinated effort. In an institution, this includes the involvement of staff extending from the highest level of administration to housekeeping. It includes nursing, medicine, pharmacy, and physiotherapy. It includes the maintenance workers, such as the carpenters and the electricians, and it includes administration, such as the Vice President for Nursing, area supervisors, risk management, and quality assurance staff. Unfortunately, it may even involve the legal department.

The concern of patients who fall is not confined to nursing, and nurses at the bedside must not and cannot solely bear the brunt of responsibility—and the guilt—when patients fall. However, preventing patients' falls is a concern that may be spearheaded and coordinated by nursing, and it is an area where leadership in prevention may fall on nursing's shoulders.

There are five basic sequential steps in establishing a fall prevention program, and the program should not be implemented until all steps are in place. If one of the steps fails to materialize, then the program should not be implemented. The five steps are illustrated as a flowchart in Figure 1.2.

Step 1: Obtain administrative support. The first step is to present the plan to administration and to obtain support and some commitment of funding for the program. Briefly, the program will consist of ensuring that the environment is optimally safe for patients, details for which are outlined in Chapter 2. Most of the equipment that staff will be suggesting, such as comfortable and safe chairs, already should be available. "Renovations," such as the addition of handrails in patients' rooms, will prove invaluable in preventing falls and enhancing patient mobility.

The real cost may be in staffing: It is recommended that a clinical nurse specialist be appointed to oversee the program (in a parallel role to the "infection control nurse"), and this means creating a new position. The second major and ongoing cost will be providing extra staff to assist on floors when the program is established. When regular staff are too busy to monitor a patient closely, extra staff may be needed to protect a patient from falling. The immediate costs may be in purchasing safety equipment, such as handrails or bed alarms. However, these requests are not exorbitant nor are they extraordinary: If hospitals are to be accountable for patients' care, then having a safe wheelchair, a bed alarm, and a comfortable seat should not be considered extraordinary.

> Nurses cannot reduce fall rates alone without funding and support.

If nursing administrations, or the Vice President for Nursing, do not support the program, then *do not continue.* Nurses cannot reduce fall rates alone nor do so without funding and support. Furthermore, as mentioned in the preface, commencing a program without providing safe interventions places nurses in a helpless position. They will then know that a patient most probably will fall, yet they do not have the supports needed to prevent the fall. The only alternative is

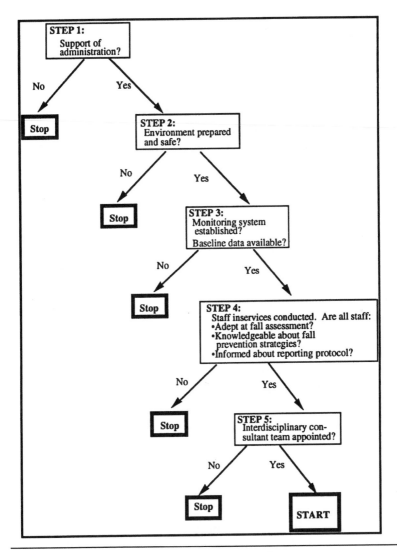

STEP 1:
Support of administration?

No → **Stop**

Yes →

STEP 2:
Environment prepared and safe?

No → **Stop**

Yes →

STEP 3:
Monitoring system established?
Baseline data available?

No → **Stop**

Yes →

STEP 4:
Staff inservices conducted. Are all staff:
• Adept at fall assessment?
• Knowledgeable about fall prevention strategies?
• Informed about reporting protocol?

No → **Stop**

Yes →

STEP 5:
Interdisciplinary consultant team appointed?

No → **Stop**

Yes → **START**

Figure 1.2. Process of Preparing to Implement a Fall Prevention Program

unacceptable and that is to restrain the patient—a procedure that will cause harm and further deterioration of the patient's condition.

Step 2: Conduct an environmental safety check. Once administration has agreed to support the program, the next step is to conduct a check of each unit to ensure that the environment is safe. This action will minimize the likelihood of accidental falls, and because patients will find it easier to ambulate—and to ambulate with more confidence—then they will become stronger (and less likely to experience a physiological fall). Because patients are able to ambulate more safely without nursing assistance, there will be some conservation of staff time.

The newly appointed clinical nurse specialist should work through each unit systematically at this time, negotiating with staff which equipment should go for repair, where railings should be installed, and what other furniture or equipment should be purchased or replaced. Until these modifications and repairs have been completed, the program must not commence.

Step 3: Obtain baseline data. The third step is to collect statistics on the number of patient falls in the institution before the fall prevention program begins, and this step may be conducted concurrently with the second step. These preintervention statistics are important because they will tell you (a) how serious the problem of patient falls is (and therefore help you justify the cost of a prevention program), and (b) how effective the program has been for reducing falls. Thus, to assess the efficacy of the program, pretest data must be available for comparison. Available statistics must be checked and compiled so that comparisons may be made readily.

Step 4: Establish a monitoring system. Often, when a fall prevention program begins, the sudden focus on falls changes nurses' reporting habits: Reporting falls is no longer perceived to be a "punishment." Suddenly, "Why did *I* let this patient fall?" becomes "Why didn't this intervention work?" and the removal of blame from the nurse and the change in attitude results in a change of reporting norms. Nurses suddenly report *all* falls, so that the fall rate unexpectedly increases dramatically. Thus, a useful check is to also prepare comparison statistics on the *injury rate* for all injuries that will have been reported. Although injuries form a less likely occurrence—and therefore longer periods have to be compared (such as year by year)—they form a more reliable indicator of the value of the program. In addition, it is

prevention of injury that is the ultimate goal of the program. A system for recording the patient's fall score in the patient's chart or Kardex needs to be developed. In addition, because the patient who falls is highly likely to fall again at the same time and under the same circumstances, a system of recording details of each fall must be developed (such as recording all falls in a notebook), and this record should be kept on the unit. A system of recording and compiling hospitalwide statistics should be developed so that there is an ongoing check of the fall-prone patients and the high-risk fall areas.

Finally, in conjunction with quality assurance and nursing administration, decisions need to be made about how and when to score each patient and how these scores will be recorded. Most important, decisions need to be made for each area about the score that will result in the patient being labeled "at risk of falling," and when fall prevention strategies will be implemented. It is important to note that with the Morse Fall Scale, for example, this score may be 16 for medium risk and 25 for high risk on a medical-surgical unit, and 25 for medium risk and 45 for high risk on a geriatric unit. The methods for making these decisions are presented in Chapter 4.

Step 5: Prepare staff. By this time, the word should have reached the unit level about the program, and staff training sessions may begin. Staff in-services should be conducted in small groups and should consist of the following:

1. Identify the fall prone patient. A short video is available for using the Morse Fall Scale,[3] and this may be left on the unit for the staff to view at their convenience. Small, plastic-covered pocket cards of the Morse Fall Scale may be prepared and distributed to staff.
2. Develop a means for identifying fall prevention strategies (see Chapter 5) and the appropriate use of the bed alarms (see Chapter 2).

3. Develop a system for recording the patient's fall score.
4. Develop a system for reporting falls.
5. Develop protocol for consulting with the "fall nurse" and the falls consultation team.

Hold inservices for staff, and present the main methods of preventing falls and the institutional protocol for recording and reporting patient falls, as well as protocols for consulting with the fall prevention clinical nurse specialist. It is a smart idea to give the unit 2 weeks of practice using the Morse Fall Scale and recording their scores. In my experience, this allows the staff to become familiar with the scale and expert at fall assessment before the program formally begins.

Step 6: Appoint an interdisciplinary assessment team. The final step before commencing the program is the appointment of an interdisciplinary team. The role of the team is to combine expertise and to consult about "problem" patients who fall repeatedly or are at exceptionally high risk of falling. The team should also periodically review all fall reports, looking particularly for institutional patterns. For example, the team may observe that many falls occur in a particular place and may be able to identify a handrail or some other structural modification that will increase the safety of the area. The team should be chaired by the fall prevention clinical nurse specialist and should be composed of the patient's primary nurse, a geriatrician, a physical therapist, a pharmacist, and an occupational therapist. Ad hoc members may include the patient (if oriented) or the patient's next-of-kin, and the patient's physician.

At the unit level, cases may be reviewed by nursing staff, with the fall prevention clinical nursing specialist serving as a consultant. Note that the goal of the consultation is to develop a plan to reduce the patient's fall risk score, to develop strategies to prevent a fall, or, if a fall has occurred, to try to develop unique and individualized strategies to prevent a recurrence. Once these things are in place, the program can begin.

Notes

1. Throughout this book, I have used the term *patient* to refer to a patient or a resident, regardless of setting.

2. Some authors sort falls into *intrinsic* and *extrinsic* causes (Morris & Isaacs, 1980). Intrinsic factors are those caused by the patient's illness or condition, such as a stroke or an amputation. Extrinsic factors are those caused by the environment, such as factors causing the patient to slip or trip.

3. Copies of the training video are available from the Glenrose Rehabilitation Hospital, 10230 -111 Avenue, Edmonton, Alberta T5G 0B7, Canada.

2

Creating a Safe Environment

Preventing Accidental Falls

Ensuring a safe environment will minimize the number of accidental falls in an institution. A safe environment will also reduce the number of potential lawsuits against the institution, thus indirectly saving staff time and preserving staff morale. It will also build staff morale because staff will recognize that administration supports their goals for a fall-prevention program. In this chapter, I will discuss the ideal environment for fall prevention and environmental features that will facilitate patient mobility and safety and ensure safe equipment.

Ensuring a Safe Environment

Hospital units are not designed for patients, to enhance patient mobility, or to prevent falls. Rather, hospital environments are designed for the staff and for the ease of moving equipment, such as beds or wheelchairs. This is not to argue that it is not possible to make the environment safer for a patient with a weak or impaired gait to mobilize, rather that funding will certainly help.

Structural Features as a Threat to Patient Safety

In hospitals, the patient's room has been designed to permit the gurney (i.e., stretcher) through the door and to fit on either side of the bed so that the patient may be transferred safely either onto or off the bed. Unfortunately, hospital doorways have been built twice the width of domestic doorways. In addition, the bed may be in the center of the room, with no hand support for the patient to grasp when climbing out of bed—except for the bedside locker, also on wheels. The patient's weakness resulting from illness or surgery itself is compounded by bed rest, so that to the patient, it seems a very long way to the bathroom. A serious concern is that often there are no handrails on the walls. Should patients fall and hurt themselves on the furniture, the staff paradoxically have cleared the room of all extraneous furniture that could be used for support.

When patients with a weak or impaired gait move about their room, they use the furniture for support, and the position of the furniture determines the route they must take. When a gap in the supportive furniture occurs, the patient looks for the next support, takes several small steps, and "dives," arms outstretched, for the next support.

This diving is particularly dangerous for the elderly. Failing eyesight, diminishing coordination, and the extra distance, for example, that it takes to cross a doorway in the hospital result in what we call the "Wonderland phenomena," named from the description of Alice's experiences in *Through the Looking Glass,* when everything appears larger as she becomes smaller. Spatial disorientation frequently occurs when the newly admitted patient has not learned the different dimensions of the hospital environment.

The solution to this problem is to create a safe path with supports for the patient to use between the bed and the bathroom. First, and

Have handrails installed in the patients' rooms and on all walls between the bed and the bathroom.

most important, have handrails installed in the patients' rooms and on all walls between the bed and the bathroom. Because this is the region where most falls occur, and such rails may prevent or break a fall and therefore prevent injury, they are worth the investment. Ideally, these rails should be round so that they may provide the optimal grip.

Flat handrails, while serving the dual purpose of protecting the walls from damage with gurneys and other carts, force the patient to hold with a pinch grip, and this position of the hand is less effective than gripping a round rail (Holliday, Fernie, Maki, & Lauzon, 1985). Handrails should be installed at an appropriate height, approximately 31 inches (.97 m or less) from the floor (see Maki, Bartlett, & Fernie, 1985).

Floors

Linoleum floors in the institution should be sealed with a matte, nonglare polish. A shiny finish blinds elderly residents with poor visual accommodation. If the sun shines through windows and creates a glare (particularly down corridors), then install venetian blinds to block the sunshine. Many institutions are now using low pile carpets that may be cleaned. Although carpeting provides more traction for the patient's feet when climbing out of bed, if the patient has an impaired gait and *slides* his or her feet along the floor when walking (i.e., the patient is not strong enough to lift his or her feet), then carpeting is likely to drag on the patient's slippers, thus contributing to a fall. Slippers with a smooth sole may, in part, relieve this problem, but those slippers then lack traction needed on tile and linoleum floors.

Comfortable Seating

Because it is poor care to keep elderly patients sitting upright in wheelchairs all day, the unit must have safe, comfortable seating for elderly patients. Recliners (with a waterproof seat cover) are ideal because the patients may lie back and have their feet raised when they wish to rest, and patients do not slide out of these chairs as easily as they tend to do from a geriatric chair. Hospital-grade beanbag chairs are ideal for patients who are restless, and make chair restraints (such as a Posey® belt or a geri-chair with a locked tray) unnecessary.

Safe Area for Wandering Patients

One of the reasons for the use of restraints is that many hospitals do not provide an enclosed area for confused and wandering patients to walk. This area should be supervised; it should contain comfortable chairs, a large space for pacing, long areas with handrails for patients who need that support when walking, a table for activities, large bright windows, and bathroom facilities.

If a separate area is not available for wandering patients, or if the staff are afraid the patient will wander at night, an alarm system to alert nursing staff when a patient is leaving the area may be a feasible option.

These alarms take two forms. The first type consists of a sensor worn by the patient and sensors installed in the doorways out of the unit (such as *No Go* alarm). When the patient tries to leave the area, the sensor on the patient triggers the door alarm and alerts the staff, who may then guide the patient back into the unit.

The second type consists of alarms on the exit door that sound when the door is opened (such as the *Tether Alarm®*). Whereas these alarms are excellent for home use, where they may be used to alert sleeping family members, in an institution they are most useful if installed on an individual patient's room door so that the nurse may be alerted if the patient tries to leave the room.

Note that door alarms are useful only in preventing patients from wandering from the unit. If the patient scores at high risk of falling, then a bed or chair alarm should be used so that nursing staff may assist the patient in getting out of bed, getting up from the chair, and ambulating.

Alternative methods for "securing" patients in an area to wander exist. For instance, the door to the area could be fitted with two door handles about 12 inches apart (that the cognitively impaired would have difficulty opening) or a "baffle latch" (Brungardt, 1994). Fabric strips may be placed across the door and fastened with Velcro to remind the wandering patient not to exit. Units must consider other solutions as well, such as using volunteers or family members to sit with patients to discourage their wandering behaviors.

Beds

The patient's bed should be high-low adjustable so that caregivers may raise the bed to provide care without causing back injuries to themselves when they try to lift a patient. It should be an electric bed, with the controls for the backrest within the patient's reach so that the backrest is adjustable by the patient. When the bed is in a low position, the mattress height (i.e., the height of the top surface of the mattress) should not be higher than a domestic bed (i.e., 16 inches), so that when a patient of average height is sitting on the bed, both feet should be flat on the floor. The patient should not have to "jump" to reach the floor when getting out of bed, nor should he or she have to use a footstool. When getting into bed, the patient should be able to get in by sitting on the side of the bed and then lying back while lifting the legs; patients should never have to get into bed by climbing in, as though climbing up a cliff! When the brake is on, the bed should not move at all—a person should be able to lean against the bed without it sliding, either by skidding on its brakes or slipping on the floor. Preferably, when the bed is in low position, the bed locks automatically. For transporting the patient, the perfect bed requires that the wheels "kick in" or the bed be raised slightly off the floor. Finally, when moving, the wheels should not "shimmy"—they should be steady, and the bed should travel around corners easily.

Step Stools

Step stools are often provided to assist patients in climbing onto (or off of) a bed or an examination table. They may be necessary if the bed or examining table is too high to otherwise reach, but caregivers must not forget that stepstools are dangerous. The risk is highest when the patient is climbing down from the bed, when it is necessary to place both feet on the stool and then step onto the floor. Because of the risk of falling off of the step stool, it is recommended that patients are always assisted when using the step stool.

Side Rails

The patient's bed should be equipped with three-quarter length side rails. *Full-length side rails are dangerous* because to exit the bed, the patient must either climb over the top of the rail (thus gaining an extra 14 inches height to fall) or climb over the end of the bed, thus falling over a "vertical cliff." If the side rails are three-quarter length, the patient has an exit route and may slide relatively safely from the bed, using the side rail as a hand hold. Furthermore, the time required to scoot down to the end of the bed gives bed alarms time to sound warning and for staff to move to the room to assist the patient.

> Side rails must not be used as a restraint.

Bed Alarms

Bed alarms are used to alert staff that a patient is getting out of bed. They provide an audible alarm when the patient moves toward the foot of the bed or tries to stand beside the bed. Some beds have an alarm system installed in the bed itself; other alarms consist of a separate sensor that is placed under the patient and is connected to a sensor unit and also may be connected to the emergency or nurse call bell system.

A common portable alarm is the pressure-sensitive strip alarm that may be placed beneath the patient's sheet about the level of the patient's buttocks. It is attached to an alarm unit that is placed on the patient's side rails and connected to a power supply. The alarm sounds when the patient's weight is removed from the strip. The alarm sounds with a delay of 4 to 9 seconds at a preset number of seconds so that false alarms do not occur with the patient turning in bed. The main disadvantage of these alarms is that if the patient is agile, the patient may be out of bed before the nurse can reach the bedside to assist the patient. Because most of the falls are *from* the bed, it is important that an alarm system be developed that will sense the patient's movements before the patient is at risk of falling.

Chair Alarms

There are several types of chair alarms that may be used to alert nursing staff when a patient attempts to get out of a chair.

1. The *Bed Check Alarm®* consists of disposable pressure-sensitive strips that are placed on the seat of the chair along with an alarm unit that is clipped onto the back of the chair. The alarm sounds after a preset number of seconds after the patient has risen from the chair.
2. The *Ambularm®* consists of an alarm unit that is worn on a garter above the patient's knee and sounds when the patient stands.
3. The *Tether Alarm®* works when a connection from the patient to the alarm becomes disconnected when the patient stands.

These patients must be carefully observed. Because all of these alarms are activated when the patient stands, it is important that they are not used with patients with an impaired gait, or with patients who cannot bear weight.

Wheelchairs

Wheelchairs become a safety hazard when they are poorly main-tained. The footrests should easily fold out of the patient's way when the patient tries to stand, and they should not flop down and interfere with the patient's standing. The brakes should be easily applied, secure (i.e., hold the chair steady as the patient stands), and easily released.

Wheelchairs tip under certain circumstances: If the patient has the legs up, and the patient is in plaster casts, then the chair is likely to be unbalanced and prone to tip forward, and anti-tip devices should be installed. The back of the chair should be weighted. Patients should be taught to manage the back tip, but antitip devices also should be installed to prevent the chair from falling backwards.

Chairs

First of all, patients' chairs should be comfortable. Often, institutional concerns for hygiene result in vinyl-covered chairs that are easy to slide out of. Chairs should have a wide seat, perhaps sloping slightly backwards. They should have a side base, and they should be heavy enough to rise from without sliding backwards. The arms should be sturdy because they are often used as a leverage to push against when getting out of the chair.

Conducting Equipment Safety Checks

In many institutions, although most equipment considered to place the patient at risk (such as incubators and elevators) is checked on a regular basis by qualified staff, the equipment used daily, such as wheelchairs, is not checked on a regular schedule. Most institutions appear to rely on nursing staff and other users to request repairs when needed. Unfortunately, because most units do not have spare wheelchairs to replace those being sent for repairs, and as necessary repairs are postponed, unsafe equipment remains in circulation.

> Check all equipment with maintenance personnel.

A check of equipment on the unit should be undertaken initially with the maintenance person in charge of repairs. Start at one end of the unit and tag equipment that does not pass with a sticker (dated). The major areas to be checked for safety are listed in Table 2.1.

Table 2.1 Equipment Checklist

Equipment Safety Checklist

Wheelchairs
  Brakes   Secure chair when on?   ____
  Arm rest   Detach easily for transfer bar?   ____
  Leg rest   Easily adjusted?   ____
  Foot pedals   Fold easily so that patient may stand?   ____
  Wheels   Are not bent or warped?   ____
  Anti-tip devices   Installed?   ____

IV stands
  Pole   Raises and lowers easily?   ____
  Wheels   Roll easily and turn freely, do not stick?   ____
  Stability   Will not tip over easily? (should be a five-point base)   ____

Beds
  Side rails   Raise and lower easily?   ____
                      Secure when up?   ____
  Wheels   Roll/turn easily, do not stick?   ____
  Brakes   Secure bed when on?   ____

Footstools
  Legs   Rubber skid protectors on all feet?   ____
                      Steady—do not rock?   ____
  Top   Nonskid surface?   ____

Call bells
  Working?   Light outside door?   ____
                      Buzzer sounds?   ____
                      Alarms in nursing station?   ____
                      Intercom satisfactory?   ____
                      Accessible in bathrooms?   ____
                      Cord pulls in good condition?   ____
                      Room panel signals working?   ____

Walkers
  Secure   Rubber tips in good condition?   ____
                      Unit stable?   ____

Canes
  Secure   Rubber tips in good condition?   ____

Commodes
  Wheels   Roll/turn easily, do not stick?   ____
                      Are weighted and not "top heavy" when a patient
                        is sitting on it?   ____

Geri-chairs
  Wheels   Roll/turn easily, do not stick?   ____
                      Brakes secure when on?   ____
  Tray   Secure?   ____

It is important that the safety check be repeated at regular intervals and the responsibility for conducting the survey assigned to a particular staff member. It is not something that is simply done once and then forgotten.

Patient Safety Care Practices

Ideally, nurses learn to routinely protect patients from hazardous situations, thereby preventing falls. For example, placing the call bell within reach is taught to nurses as a routine part of patient care from the first clinical experience. Nurses recognize that when reaching for a call bell, patients may lose balance and fall from the bed or a chair. Furthermore, a call bell that is out of reach is also "out of mind." In particular, elderly patients may forget how to call the nurse, and when actual calling (i.e., shouting) fails to bring help, he or she may try to get out of bed unassisted, thereby risking a fall.

> The most frequently cited cause of falls is "going to the bathroom unassisted."

Similarly, personal belongings and things that are needed often, such as a water glass, should be in easy reach of the bed. Make sure that the patient's bedside stand is within reach, and each time the nurse is with the patient, he or she should check that the patient has everything he or she needs.

The most frequently cited cause of falls is "going to the bathroom unassisted." Not only does this involve the risk of getting out of bed unassisted, but the patient, who is hoping that help will arrive, also may wait until the last minute to go and thus is frequently in a hurry. Urinary urgency and frequency add to the patient's haste, and, if incontinent, patients have slipped in their urine. Good nursing care includes regular toileting of patients, especially at night. Patients should be checked routinely and regularly to see if they have any other needs, and they should be allowed to exercise or walk at least three times a day.

Safe, nonskid, well-fitting slippers are important. Patients often arrive in hospital with new but impractical and unsafe slippers. They may be scuffs or have slippery soles. Similarly, ill-fitting, disposable, hospital slippers made from foam are also impractical for walking—especially if the patient has an impaired gait—and should not be used.

Long bathrobes or female patients' long nightgowns that reach the floor are very dangerous because the patient may tread on the hem and fall. This hazard may become more problematic if the patient has had abdominal surgery and walks with a stooped gait, attempting to protect the wound and prevent pain. Hospital gowns that open at the back and secure with two or three ties also create a fall risk because the patient may lose his or her balance when walking, attempting to preserve modesty by holding the gown closed in back. The best solution is to give the patient two gowns to wear over each other, with one tied at the back and one tied at the front.

The night lighting must be bright enough for the patient to become quickly oriented on waking and to remember where he or she is. Night lighting also must be bright enough for patients to find their bedside lighting and call bell, to find their slippers and gown, to find their way safely to the bathroom without falling over or walking into anything, and to find the bathroom light switches. Night lights that provide a reasonable glow and are set close to the floor are a good solution: Bright lights that shine into a room from a bathroom or hallway may be so bright as to interfere with sleep or may temporarily blind the patient on waking.

3

Monitoring Falls in the Institution

Monitoring falls, the injuries resulting from falls, and the eventual outcome is crucial. Monitoring provides the means to inform the nurses and the administration of the seriousness of the problem of falls and the effectiveness of the fall prevention program. The regular reporting of the fall rates of each unit as well as the total institution to staff motivates them to continue their fall prevention efforts and provides them with the satisfaction of seeing the incidence of falls—and of serious injuries—decline.

Recording Fall Rates

Defining a Fall

Unfortunately, there is no clear definition of a fall. Morris and Isaacs (1980) defined it as an event in which the patient came to rest on the floor. Therefore, this definition includes patients who slipped from a chair onto the floor, perhaps includes patients who were found lying on the floor (but were not actually seen falling), and includes falls in which a bystander caught the patient (and therefore broke the impact of the fall) but in which the patient was lowered to the floor. But clearly, this definition does not include instances in which the patients have fallen but managed to flop down onto a bed or into a chair. Nor does it include a slip in a bathtub, or many other occurrences that could be listed. And the definition does not include patients who fell and were not found but managed to get up unassisted. Thus, in some instances, it is very clear when a patient falls or has fallen, but in other instances, it is not so clear. Compounding the problem is that patients who are prone to falling are very often poor historians regarding a fall. They may not consider a slip or a trip a *real* fall, they may forget to report the fall, or they may be too embarrassed to mention the event to a staff member.

Exactly what constitutes a fall is therefore left to the best judgment of the staff member. However, it is important to note that if the fall prevention program is going to reduce falls, the goal is to prevent all falls, *including the first fall.* Therefore, if a staff member *prevents* a fall, say, by catching a patient, then this should be noted in the patient's record because a "missed fall" is a piece of useful information for improving a fall prevention strategy.

How to Measure the Incidence of Falls

There are a number of methods to measure the incidence of falls in an institution, and these methods are not equivalent. It is recommended that institutions select and report their incidence of falls using the *fall rate.* The fall rate is the most reliable method because it includes *all falls* in its calculation, not just the number of patients *who have fallen,* so that although a patient who falls repeatedly may apparently artificially inflate the statistics, it is an accurate reflection of the number of times a patient is actually at risk of injury. The fall rate also is calculated on the number of *patient bed days,* rather than the number of patients at risk, which does not consider the length of stay.

The *fall rate* may be calculated using the following formula:

$$\frac{\text{number of patient falls}}{\text{number of patient bed days}} \times 1,000$$

However, because the formula is not restricted to a particular time frame, for future reference state the period for which the statistics were collected. One warning, however, when using the above formula: When a fall prevention program is initiated, there is often a change of attitude in the staff. Previously, it may have been a nuisance to complete a fall report form when a patient fell, or nurses may have considered falls to be an indicator of poor care and a reason for self-blame; now, however, interest in falls that comes with a prevention program suddenly makes it acceptable to have a resident fall. The attitude shifts from "Why did I let this patient fall?" to "Why didn't this strategy work?" This removal of personal responsibility from the incident results in an increase in reporting of resident falls, which in turn results in an artificial fluctuation in the fall rate. Just when the fall rate should be decreasing, the change in reporting of falls results in an artificial increase in the fall rate.

To calculate the *patient fall rate*, suppose an institution collected the following statistics:

Number of patient falls (1986 calendar year)   147
Number of patient bed days (1986 calendar year)   49,946

Using these data, the *fall rate* for the institution for 1986 may be calculated as follows:

$$\frac{147}{49,946} \times 1,000 = 2.9 \text{ falls per 1,000 patient bed days}$$

However, not all institutions, or all research articles, use this statistic. Other institutions may report such statistics as the *number of patients at risk*, the *number of patients who fell*, the *number of falls per bed*, and the *probability of falling*. A comparison of methods for calculating fall rates are presented in Appendix D.

The Injury Rate

The *injury rate* is an indirect measure of the fall rate because one may argue that it is, in part, a matter of chance whether or not a patient is injured when he or she falls. For instance, it is a matter of chance if a piece of furniture was present on which the patient hit his or her head and sustained an injury. However, as staff more reliably complete an incident report form when an injury occurs, and because it is really the *injuries* that are problematic, the injury rate provides an important indicator monitoring institutional falls.

The *injury rate* may be calculated as follows:

$$\frac{\text{number of patients injured}}{\text{number of patients who fell}} \times 100 \text{ per time period}$$

To avoid artificially inflating the statistic, be sure to include only *one injury per patient.* For instance, if a patient fractured an arm and a hip in the same fall, count that as *one* injury. In addition, when demonstrating the efficacy of a fall prevention program, it may be helpful to the institution to calculate the rate of *minor, moderate,* and *major* injuries separately. For example, in a trial to test the efficacy of the Morse Fall Scale at Veterans Affairs Medical Center, Portland, Oregon (see McCollam, 1995), the fall rate increased 24% (perhaps because of changes in reporting norms and including near-falls in the calculation), but the number of serious injuries from falls fell 174% to an all-time low of four falls. The injury rate, however, was not reported.

Classifying Injuries

Classifying the degree of injury is important for purposes of analysis. Although it is relatively easy to classify injuries into two or three categories (usually minor and serious, or minor, moderate, and major), it is important that the criteria for classification are published so that others

---

Use a standardized method of classifying injury.

Table 3.1 Classification of Severity of Injury

No Injury:	No evidence of abrasion or bruising and no complaint of pain following the fall.
Minor:	Any small bruise or abrasion that does not require medical treatment and will heal within several days.
Moderate:	Injury requiring medical treatment that is not considered major. For example, a small cut that requires only a few sutures, or an IV that infiltrates and needs to be reinserted. Bruises and contusions are considered moderate if they require treatment, and sprains as well as suspected bone injury are considered moderate if an X ray is ordered and there is no fracture.
Major:	A serious injury, including any fracture, head injury, or wound that requires major suturing.

may compare their data. At present, there is a confusing array of classifications. Some authors have included only fractures in the "major" category, whereas others have included head injuries (such as a concussion), soft tissue injury that required suturing, and fractures. It is recommended that the classification system shown in Table 3.1 be used when classifying the degree of injury.

A second problem that occurs when using the injury rate is that injuries often are not diagnosed for several days after the incident. For instance, after an elderly patient falls, a minor injury, such as a bruised hip, may be reported. However, when the patient continues to complain of pain several days after the incident, an X-ray may be ordered and a hairline fracture of the pelvis diagnosed. In these cases, it is important to correct the original fall report form. It is therefore recommended that administrative follow-up of injuries be conducted routinely approximately 4 days after the fall and that seriously injured patients be followed until the consequences and outcome of their falls and injuries are known. In many instances, the eventual outcome of a fractured hip in an elderly patient is death weeks or months after

Routinely follow up patients 4 days after the fall to ensure that injuries have not been subsequently diagnosed.

the incident. These outcomes, however, are usually not included in the incident report form nor noted by the administration.

Common Errors in Reporting

Because a number of methods are used to report patient falls, it is often difficult to compare the fall rate between institutions, between patient populations, and/or when evaluating fall prevention programs. Usually, the length of time in which data were collected is not reported, and readers frequently are unable to ascertain if repeated falls (which are dependent events) have been included in the calculations. Because there are difficulties with most of the methods used, it is recommended that the fall rate (i.e., the number of falls/number of patient bed days × 1,000) be used as a standard measure. Other statistics, such as the *number of patients at risk*, the *number of repeated falls*, and the *number of patients injured*, should be reported so that all necessary calculations and comparisons can be made. And finally, if, after implementing a fall prevention program, the expected reduction in *fall rates* does not occur, administrators should examine all possible reasons for failure, including changes in staffing levels, patient acuity, and reporting norms.

> To reduce error, use the fall rate as a standard measure.

Establishing Baseline Data

Before embarking on a fall prevention program, administration must ascertain whether or not a fall prevention program is needed and how serious the problem of patient falls is. Thus, the first step is to use available data from hospital statistics to create a table to illustrate the incidence of falls for as many years as possible. Examine the fall rate for each year as well as the injury rate. Compare these rates—were they consistent over the years? From these, it will be possible to ascertain how serious the problem of patient falls is in the institution, and following the implementation of the program, these statistics will provide the evidence necessary to show the reduction of the fall rate and the injury rate, as well as to justify the cost of the fall prevention program.

Institutional Monitoring

Deciding What to Count

In Chapter 1, the ambiguity of exactly what a fall is was discussed. Often, it is clear that the patient has fallen because the nurse may observe the fall or hear the thud as the patient hits the floor. But if a patient slips and prevents him- or herself from falling by grabbing the handrail, does that near-fall count in the statistics? If a patient is at the end of the bed and found (and caught) by a nurse as he or she is about to fall, that is a prevented fall—a near miss—a successfully prevented fall, but the actual fall did not occur.

When deciding on the efficacy of a program, in addition to counting the actual falls, the administration may also decide to count the "near misses"—the prevented falls—as an additional indicator of success of the program. The prevented falls could be listed separately and noted by the unit. Not only are they a means to provide credit to the nurses who prevented the incident, but they provide additional data about the patient's fall risk; the time, place, and context of possible falls; and possible future recurrence.

How to Record

Staff routinely record information about a fall on an incident report form. These forms provide information about the patient's activity and events surrounding the fall. The form provides information about any witnesses, as well as the time, date, and activity at the time the fall occurred. The form also should have a record on how many previous falls the patient has had, and it should contain space to list the patient's Morse Fall Scale total score and scores for each item. Incident report forms provide information about any injury and treatments required and whether the family and physicians were notified of the fall. These forms are then placed in the patient's chart, and a carbon copy is forwarded to Risk Management and to the Fall Clinical Nurse Specialist. The Fall Clinical Nurse Specialist then conducts a fall assessment and schedules a conference on the patient with the multidisciplinary team. The fall must also be recorded on the patient's chart and noted in the unit's fall log record.

The fall log record consists of a listing of each patient who falls, where the fall occurred, the patient activity at the time of the fall, and the time the fall occurred. Each patient should be listed in a separate section, for if a subsequent fall occurs, as mentioned in Chapter 6, the fall log record will aid in identifying patterns of falls and help prevent recurrence of falls.

Responsibility for Monitoring

The person whose primary responsibility is to monitor patient falls is the Fall Clinical Nurse Specialist. It is his or her responsibility to collate the fall statistics, coordinate the fall consultation team, provide feedback to the patient's primary nurse, and ensure that all shifts are aware of the special fall prevention strategies developed for certain patients. The Fall Clinical Nurse Specialist must prepare monthly reports on the number of falls and the number and type of injuries, both for the institution and for each unit. These reports also should show the statistics for the previous month and for the same period the previous year. This feedback to staff is vital because it aids in demonstrating to the staff that all of their prevention efforts are worthwhile. However, recall that the fall rate will increase over the period prior to the initiation of the program because of changes in reporting norms.

4

Predicting *Physiological Anticipated Falls*

The nursing approach is based on the underlying assumption that falls should not occur if the care is excellent, and it places considerable responsibility on the individual staff member and, consequently, on the institution. For example, Arsenault (1982) writes:

> "It could have happened to any of us!" These words keep reverberating in my head as I remember my return to work after an eight day vacation.
>
> It was a calm Saturday evening. Mr. Smith was one of my five patients. He was an elderly man admitted to the hospital for treatment of an aspirate pneumonia. He was physically improving, but he continued to have diarrhea secondary to Iscal tube feedings. To prevent fecal incontinence, Mr. Smith routinely used his commode unattended before he retired to bed. So I left him on his commode [while I left] to care for another patient. This evening, Mr. Smith never did make it back to bed. Five minutes later I was summoned to

his room. . . . There he lay—ashen, unresponsive and bleeding from
a gash in his head. He had fallen while attempting to walk to the
bathroom. Mr. Smith died two weeks later. (p. 386)

Thus, even if the fall was primarily caused by the patient's underlying
medical condition, nurses apparently feel that it is their responsibility
to *prevent any fall from occurring.*

Assessing Fall Risk

Patient Assessment

Because of diverse perspectives on the reasons underlying patient
falls, there are basically three types of scales or instruments available
to assist in identifying the patient who falls. The first group consists
of scales that separate the patients who may fall from those who may
not and *predict the likelihood* of a patient fall, so that fall prevention
strategies and resources may be targeted to the patients most likely to
fall and, therefore, *prevent* the patient from falling. These forms are
short, quick, and easy to use and are intended to be used at least once
daily.

The second group, *fall assessment forms,* assists staff in identifying
the possible causes of falls. These forms usually consist of some form
of environmental checks (such as bed in the low position), patient behaviors (patient gait, confusion), nursing care strategies (toilet patient
regularly, remind patient to use call bell), possible problems in the
medical regimen (number of medications), and prevention strategies
("reinforce fall risk with families"). These forms are long and cumbersome and are intended to be used once, usually on admission.

The third type is intended to be used *after the patient has fallen.*
These forms consist of a space to write details of the fall itself,
including the patient's account of the incident, patient behavior at the
time the incident occurred, and any injures sustained; a physical
examination checklist to record the patient's condition; and any
recommendation for prevention in the future. These forms are also

long and cumbersome and are intended to be completed by the physician, nurse practitioner, or physical therapist.

As mentioned previously, it is important that when selecting a method of assessing patient falls, the instrument should be used as the researcher has published it. Changing any of the items or the item scores destroys the reliability and validity of the scale and may even result in the scale losing its ability to predict falls. Similarly, although it is tempting to "improve" these scales by creating your own—for instance, by selecting the apparent "best" items from several scales—such measures may result in a scale with no reliability or validity. Use a scale in its entirety, and select a scale that has reported reliability and validity.

The Morse Fall Scale

The Morse Fall Scale is a rapid and simple method of assessing a patient's likelihood of falling. It consists of six variables that are quick and easy to score, and it has been shown to have predictive validity and interrater reliability.[1]

Method of Scale Construction

Patients who fell ($n = 100$) and 100 randomly selected controls were examined using a comprehensive physical examination form, inspection of environmental contributing factors, patient report of the fall, and outcome (including patient injuries). Significant variables that differentiated the patients who fell from the patients who did not fall were identified using techniques of discriminant analysis and data reduction. Scale weights were obtained for each significant variable (item), and, using techniques of computer modeling, the scale was tested on a simulated patient population. Validity was established further by splitting the data set randomly and repeating the procedures used to obtain the significant variables, and then testing them on the remaining 50% of these data. (See Appendix B.)

Examination of False Positives

The charts of 22 patients who had fallen and who were not classified as fall prone by the Morse Fall Scale were examined. This analysis showed that all patients were oriented. Despite the fact that eight patients had a weak gait, only one used a walking aid. These patient falls were classified as "unanticipated falls."

Prospective Testing

Sixteen patient care units from three types of patient care units (i.e., acute medical and surgical, long-term geriatric care, and rehabilitation areas) from two institutions used the Morse Fall Scale for a 4-month period. Daily rating of all patients resulted in 2,689 patients examined for fall score and a subsequent fall. Examination of scores in the acute care institution by length of stay revealed different patterns of fall risk; the mean score of the long-term patients showed less variation and higher scores. Analysis of patients who fell by type of fall (anticipated, unanticipated, and accidental) and the severity of injuries increased with the higher scores, indicating clinical validity of the scale (see Appendix E).

Scoring the Morse Fall Scale

Testing in the clinical area by nurses who used the scale as a part of their normal workday showed that the Morse Fall Scale is quick and easy to use. A large majority of the nurses (82.9%) rated the scale as "quick and easy to use," and 54% estimated that it took less than 3 minutes to rate a patient.

The items in the scale (see Table 4.1) are scored as follows:

History of falling. This is scored as 25 if the patient has fallen during the present hospital admission or if there was an immediate history of physiological falls, such as from seizures or an impaired gait prior to admission. If the patient has not fallen, this is scored 0. *Note:* If a patient falls for the first time, then his or her score immediately increases by 25.

Table 4.1 Morse Fall Scale

Item		Score
1. History of falling	no 0	
	yes 25	_____
2. Secondary diagnosis	no 0	
	yes 15	_____
3. Ambulatory aid		
None/bed rest/nurse assist	0	
Crutches/cane/walker	15	
Furniture	30	_____
4. Intravenous therapy/heparin lock	no 0	
	yes 20	_____
5. Gait		
Normal/bed rest/wheelchair	10	
Weak	20	
Impaired	20	_____
6. Mental status		
Oriented to own ability	0	
Overestimates/forgets limitations	15	_____
Total		_____

Secondary diagnosis. This is scored as 15 if more than one medical diagnosis is listed on the patient's chart; if not, score 0.

Ambulatory aids. This is scored as 0 if the patient walks without a walking aid (even if assisted by a nurse), uses a wheelchair, or is on bed rest and does not get out of bed at all. If the patient uses crutches, a cane, or a walker, this item scores 15; if the patient ambulates clutching onto the furniture for support, score this item 30.

Intravenous therapy. This is scored as 20 if the patient has an intravenous apparatus or a heparin lock inserted; if not, score 0.

Gait. The characteristics of the three types of gait are evident regardless of the type of physical disability or underlying cause. A *normal gait* is characterized by the patient walking with head erect, arms swinging freely at the side, and striding unhesitantly. This gait scores 0.

With a *weak gait* (score as 10), the patient is stooped but is able to lift the head while walking without losing balance. If support from furniture is required, this is with a featherweight touch almost for reassurance, rather than grabbing to remain upright. Steps are short and the patient may shuffle.

With an *impaired gait* (score 20), the patient may have difficulty rising from the chair, attempting to get up by pushing on the arms of the chair and/or by bouncing (i.e., by using several attempts to rise). The patient's head is down, and he or she watches the ground. Because the patient's balance is poor, the patient grasps onto the furniture, a support person, or a walking aid for support and cannot walk without this assistance. When assisting these patients to walk, the nurse will note that they *really* hold onto the nurse's hand, and, when grasping a rail or furniture, they often hold so that their knuckles are white. The patient takes short steps and shuffles.

If the patient is in a wheelchair, the patient is scored according to the gait he or she used when transferring from the wheelchair to the bed.

Mental status. When using the Scale, mental status is measured by checking the patient's own self-assessment of his or her own ability to ambulate. Ask the patient, "Are you able to go to the bathroom alone or do you need assistance?" If the patient's reply judging his or her own ability is consistent with the ambulatory orders on the Kardex®, the patient is rated as "normal" and scored 0. If the patient's response is not consistent with the nursing orders or if the patient's assessment is unrealistic, then the patient is considered to *overestimate his or her own abilities* and to be *forgetful of limitations* and scored as 15.

The score is then tallied and recorded on the patient's chart. It is important that none of the items on the Scale is omitted or changed. For example, some long-term care institutions may not use IV therapy. If this is the case, leave IV therapy on the Scale—it will simply always be zero for that institution. It is also important not to simplify the scores (e.g., by changing the values to single digits) because this will result in the loss of validity. For example, changing the score to 1s and 0s results in a loss of almost 30% of the number of falls correctly identified and gives a scale that predicts a fall-prone patient only slightly better than by chance. To assist nurses in remembering the items and scoring system, it is recommended that you make a small pocket card version of the Scale available to the staff.

Determining Level of Risk

The risk of falling varies greatly with different patient populations, as well as with different times of day and different stages of the patient's illness. Therefore, ideally, the Morse Fall Scale should be calibrated to each unit so that fall prevention strategies are targeted to those most at risk. This is important: Institutionwide, in an acute care hospital, the scale could be set with a high-risk cut-off score of 25. This is because in an acute care hospital, there are a lot of patients with a normal gait who are not at risk of falling. However, those who are at highest risk are "clustered" on certain units (such as the psychogeriatric unit), and if a cut-off score for high risk was set at 25 on those units, then all of the patients would score at high risk. (Of course, in some units, *all* of the patients may be at very high risk of falling, and fall prevention measures should be provided for all patients.) Thus, the high-risk score should vary according to the type of patients on the unit. Units that consist of all stroke patients, for example, will have patients who are all at risk of falling. The Scale should be set at about 45, and all patients need to be targeted for fall prevention strategies. On a surgical unit, only a few of the patients will be at very high risk of falling, and the Scale should be set at about 25.

> Calibrate the Morse Fall Scale for each particular unit so that fall prevention strategies are targeted to those most at risk.

This is very important, because if the cut-off score from a unit with a lot of disabled patients is used generally throughout the hospital, the cut-off score will be set too high. Thus, the scale will lose its sensitivity, and many of the patients who are at risk of falling will be missed (i.e., the false negative rate will increase).[2] The highest that Morse has set the scale is 45, which was in a rehabilitation hospital and a nursing home. In this case, we also targeted a medium-risk group, with scores between 35 and 44.

There are several ways to determine the cut-off score to be used. The best method is to score all of the patients in a unit and examine the distribution of these scores. In consultation with administration, the Clinical Nurse Specialist should determine the cut-off score for the percentage of patients who will be declared high risk, considering the costs of providing a fall prevention program and the benefits of the program. Examine the distribution of the scores with the scores obtained in Morse's study (Table C.1 and Table E.2) to see if the distribution of your scores on a particular unit is similar. Examine Table C.3 to see the number of patients who would be missed (considered false negatives) and the number of patients not at risk who would be considered at risk (considered false positives) and receive fall prevention for each scale score. Consultation with administration is necessary at this time because the level of high risk set for the unit has cost implications in providing fall prevention measures and may have legal implications if a patient falls and is injured, and there is a subsequent lawsuit against the hospital.

Preparing to Implement a Fall Prevention Program

Once the administrative decision has been made to invest in a fall prevention program, the structures necessary for the program must be put in place. These structures consist of appointing a clinical nurse specialist to be responsible for the implementation of the program (including providing in-service to staff) and setting up an interdisciplinary consultation team.

The Role of the Clinical Nurse Specialist

A clinical nurse specialist should be appointed as fall prevention nurse in the institution. This nurse will be responsible for setting up a recording system for fall reporting, ensuring that all staff are able to use the Morse Fall Scale reliably through in-service education, conducting fall assessment of high-risk patients and establishing fall protection regimes, conducting multidisciplinary team meetings regarding very high-risk patients and patients who fall repeatedly, providing staff with in-service education of fall prevention strategies, and meeting with relatives regarding the use (or decisions not to use) restraints. The nurse will conduct fall assessment on high-risk patients and consult with physical therapy, occupational therapy, and physicians. The nurse will do follow-up on all patients who have fallen, identify fall prevention strategies, prepare care plans accordingly, and make recommendations to prevent recurrence. He or she will track all patients who are injured in a fall to determine the impact of the injury on the patient's subsequent health and mobility levels. The nurse is also responsible for conducting (with maintenance) environmental and equipment safety checks of all units on a regular basis. Finally, he or she is responsible for the regular calculation of fall and injury rates and the reporting of these to staff and administration on a regular basis.

> A clinical nurse specialist leads the fall prevention program.

Teaching Staff

In-service instruction of all staff regarding the use of the Morse Fall Scale appears a formidable task but is not so onerous if conducted in small group sessions. Once the initial instruction is complete with the incorporation of the module into the regular staff orientation program, the use of the Scale becomes a routine and simple task. In McCollam's study (1995), the staff reported that the Scale took only

1 minute to complete and recommended that it become a part of the regular assessment forms.

A training video on the use of the Scale is available and takes 10 minutes to view. It is recommended that the Scale be reproduced on cards that the staff can carry around in their pockets and thus be prepared to refer frequently to the items on the Scale and their values.

Even if the decision has been made to score patients regularly once a day, it is important that all staff, even night staff, be familiar with and able to use the Morse Fall Scale. This is because of the variability of patients' fall risk should their conditions change. For instance, patients may be confused *only* at night (as with "sundowners"), and their judgment regarding their ability to go to the washroom unassisted at night is impaired. In such cases, the score for mental status of these patients would increase by 15 points at night, and this should be documented on the patient's chart. Alternatively, nurses may find that patients are more tired when the nurses are assisting patients back to bed, and their gait may change from weak to impaired, and their fall score should be increased accordingly. In this way, patients' fall scores may fluctuate in a 24-hour period, and the staff should be sensitive to such variability.

> All staff must be familiar with and able to use the Morse Fall Scale.

The Interdisciplinary Consultation Team

All patients who initially score at high risk of falling should be reviewed, case by case, by an interdisciplinary team. The purpose of such a review should be (a) to reduce the patient's falls score (and therefore reduce the risk of the patient falling); (b) to prevent a fall by identifying appropriate fall prevention strategies; and (c) to prevent recurrence, if the patient has fallen in the past. As mentioned in Chapter 1, the team should consist of the fall prevention clinical nurse specialist (as chairperson), the patient's primary nurse, a geriatrician, a physical therapist, a pharmacist, and an occupational therapist. Ad hoc members may include the patient (if oriented) or the patient's next-of-kin, and the patient's physician.

Notes

1. Reliability and Validity: Interrater reliability scores on the scale, using 21 raters, was $r = 0.96$. To obtain consistency, videotapes of patients' ambulating were used for this trial (Morse et al., 1989). A test for internal consistency revealed poor interitem correlation, with a coefficient alpha of .16. This, combined with the results of an analysis of variance ($F = 71.34$, $p < .00001$), suggest that the Scale items are relatively independent (see Appendix A).

Validity for the Morse Fall Scale was ensured by the method of Scale construction, examination of cases incorrectly classified by the scale (i.e., false negatives), and prospective testing of the scale to predict the fall-prone patient in three clinical settings.

2. In a recent trial of the Scale at the Veterans Affairs Medical Center, Portland, Oregon, a cut-off score of 55 was determined efficient from a pilot in a cardiology general-medical unit. This was extremely high and resulted in the loss of sensitivity of the Scale. The authors concluded that, "as suggested by Morse, cut-off scores need to be adjusted for different patient groups" (McCollam, 1995, p. 514).

5

Preventing the Fall

Once a patient has been identified as at risk of falling using the Morse Fall Scale, the task of the staff is twofold: First, to prevent the fall from occurring and second, to reduce the likelihood of the fall occurring by reducing the patient's fall score.

Remember that the Morse Fall Scale does not provide a solution for *preventing the fall*—the Scale only provides information about the likelihood of the patient falling, and the higher the score, the greater the chance of the patient falling. Furthermore, the Scale does not provide any information about *when* the patient will fall or under *what* circumstances the fall will occur. Most important, because patients fall in an infinite variety of circumstances, the interventions developed to prevent a fall cannot be standardized. Fall prevention strategies must be identified for each patient individually.

Conducting a Fall Assessment

A fall assessment should be conducted on all patients who score at risk of falling and, so that subsequent falls may be prevented, repeated after a fall occurs. Within each of the three types of falls are a myriad of factors that may cause a fall, and there are numerous strategies to prevent the fall. Identifying the cause of the fall requires observational and assessment skills of the nurse and consultation of a multidisciplinary team to identify possible physiological causes. It also requires regular checking of the environment for hazards that may have contributed to the fall. Finally, it requires developing a plan for the prevention of a subsequent fall.

Components of a Fall Assessment

Assessing the Patient's Physical Ability

This concerns the patient's ability to ambulate, to rise and get into a chair, to transfer, and to climb in and out of bed. It should also include an assessment of the patient's ability to toilet oneself—to sit on the commode and to rise from the commode and clean oneself, while managing nightgowns, robes, and pajama pants, perhaps while holding on to the support rail.

Assessing the Patient's Mental Status

Assess the patient's assessment of his or her own abilities. Is he or she able to use the call bell? Is he or she willing to ask for assistance to get up of bed, and does he or she remember to do so? Is the patient aware that he or she is unable to move about the room without support or a walking aid? Does he or she remember to use the walking aid as instructed?

Assessing the Patient's Ability and Mode of Ambulation

In the hospital, we observed that the elderly often overestimated their own abilities. In their own homes, for instance, the elderly could move about by holding onto furniture and cross doorways by reaching for the far side of the door frame. But in the hospital, this unexpectedly becomes dangerous. In hospital, the doorways are built to accommodate gurneys and therefore are wider than those in the home. There are greater distances between furniture, and it is often on wheels and slides away from the person

=====================================
Fall prevention strategies are individually planned for each patient.
=====================================

who is using it as a support. Therefore, observe how the person moves about the room. Does he or she reach for the support of furniture and "dive" across doorways reaching for the far door frame? If so, these patients must be given a walking frame to use for support and must be instructed in its use. Again, check to see if they use it consistently according to directions.

Assessing Patient's Ability to Sit

Check where the patient prefers to sit. Is the chair low and therefore difficult to rise from? On the other hand, if the patient has an impaired gait and is confused, staff may want the patient to sit in a chair that is difficult to get out of so that the patient may be easier to monitor. Is the chair comfortable? Does the chair have arms that provide adequate leverage when the patient tries to rise? Watch the patient rise. Is the patient able to rise directly, or does it take many bounces, or pushing on the arms of the chair, before the patient is upright? Is the chair stable or secure, or does it slide backwards? When the patient stands, is he or she steady, or does he or she need to reach for support immediately, even while continuing to reach back to the chair's arm rest? Does the patient grab the support and clutch onto it, or does the patient simply rest his or her fingers on that support? And when patients walk, observe their gait.

Table 5.1 Fall Prevention Strategies, According to Type of Fall

Intervention	Physiological anticipated fall	Unanticipated physiological fall[a]	Accidental fall
		Type of fall	
Identify patients with a high fall score, "flag" on chart, call light, bed, and outside the patient's door	x		
Staff unit adequately at high risk times; do not cluster all staff at report in nursing station	x		
Physician consultation	x	x	
Medication review	x	x	
Examine previous falls for patient's fall pattern	x		
Ensure patient wears eye glasses; clean them regularly	x		x
Orient patient to surroundings	x		x
Teach patient protective measures and how to anticipate falls	x	x	x
Ensure patient's footwear and clothing is an adequate fit	x		x
Assist patient ambulating	x		
Toilet patient regularly	x		
Closely observe disoriented patients; check frequently at night	x		
Ensure adequate lighting at night	x		x
Use appropriate protective devices on wheelchairs and gerichairs	x		
Monitor confused patient with bed, chair, and door alarms	x		
Keep bed in low position	x		x
Uses 3/4-length side rails	x		
Lock wheels on wheelchairs, beds, commodes, and gurneys	x		x
Wipe up spills immediately; do not polish floors	x		x
Place call bell, urinal, tissues, and water within reach	x		x
Instruct patients to call for assistance to go the bathroom	x		
Leave intercom open from patient's room to nurses' station	x		
Ensure walking aids are fitted and used appropriately	x		x
Ensure adequate exercise and PT for strengthening muscles	x		
Regularly check equipment and send for repair as necessary	x		x
Ensure appropriate hand rails in bathroom, patients' rooms, and in the hallways	x		

a. These measures may only be implemented after the first fall has occurred.

Assessing Wheelchair Use

When transferring to, rising from, or sitting down in wheelchairs, patients are at most risk of falling. Observe the patient transferring from the wheelchair to bed and vice versa. Does the patient bring the wheelchair as close as possible to the bed? Is there a height difference between the bed and the chair, and does the patient adjust the bed accordingly? Does the patient apply the brakes on the wheelchair? Is the bed braked? If the patient is weight bearing, are the leg rests and foot pedals moved out of the way so the patient can stand? Does the patient use a transfer board, and is it secure? If the patient has casts on his or her legs, is the wheelchair weighted to prevent tipping? Finally, is the wheelchair a comfortable fit considering the patient's size?

Assessing Patient's Daily Routine

Understanding the patient's routine will provide insights into the times that the patient needs assistance to go to the bathroom or when the patient may be tired, the weakest, and his or her gait most impaired. It provides important information about when the patient is awake and restless at night and for which periods during the day the patient may be most at risk and may need to be toileted or exercised. On the other hand, it provides information about the patient's patterns and times of sleep when the nurses may be less vigilant.

Assessing Patient's Need for Exercise

Patients need to be exercised, and this routine is important to prevent muscle wasting and increasing weakness. Even if the patient needs the assistance of two nurses, it is recommended that patients are regularly walked to the toilet and back to their chair rather than using a wheelchair. Establishing this routine ensures that patients are exercised as well as toileted.

Assessing Things That "Settle" the Patient

Observe the patient to ascertain to what the patient responds. What calms or settles the patient? Ask the family what type of music the patient enjoys. Ensure that patients are warm enough, because when patients are cold, they become restless.

When a Fall Occurs

When a fall occurs, the circumstances and events surrounding the fall should be recorded. Obtain as much information as possible from the patient and from witnesses about the cause of the fall. Record:

1. The circumstances surrounding the fall:
   - Where did the fall occur? Were there any environmental factors that may have contributed to the fall? Was it an accidental fall? Could a second fall be prevented by making modifications to the setting?
   - What was the patient doing at the time of the fall? Was the patient getting out of or into bed? As soon as possible, have the patient repeat the activity while you observe closely. If the patient's fall occurred while getting out of a chair, have the patient rise from the same chair. Observe if the chair was stable when the patient stood, where the patient parked his or her walker, and if the chair-walker transfer was done correctly. If the patient had to reach for the walker, consider if the patient was steady on rising and upright before beginning to walk, and so forth.
   - Was there a "warning"? Did the patient feel that he or she was going to fall, or did the patient not realize what had happened until he or she was found on the floor?
   - How did the patient fall (i.e., did the patient try to break the fall, grabbing onto something to break the fall, or was it a "free fall" without even the patient's arms breaking the impact)?
2. Determine the type of fall. According to the classification of types of falls (Chapter 1), was it an accidental, unanticipated physiological, or an anticipated physiological fall?
   - If an *accidental fall*, identify the environmental factors that may have contributed to the fall.

- If an *unanticipated physiological fall,* examine the time, the circumstances, and possible physical conditions contributing to the fall.
- If it was an *anticipated physiological fall,* examine the patient's fall score and collect information on the pattern of the fall score to determine if there is a time when the patient is more likely to be at risk of falling.

3. Meet with appropriate members of the multidisciplinary team and identify remedial fall prevention strategies to prevent the fall from recurring.

- If it was an *accidental fall,* meet with the appropriate members of the multidisciplinary team. For instance, if the fall was due to a defective wheelchair, discuss with maintenance how the system of safety checks can be improved so that all wheelchairs are included in the schedule. Develop a plan to prevent recurrence.
- If it was an *unanticipated physiological fall,* meet with the multidisciplinary team to determine how the patient's fall score may be reduced and to identify strategies to prevent recurrence. For example, if the patient was confused and was trying to get to the bathroom unassisted, review the patient's medications with the physician and the pharmacist for possible drug interactions that may contribute to the confusion. This intervention, if successful, would reduce the patient's fall score. Would preventive nursing measures, such as withholding bedtime fluids, reduce the need to void at night? Or would regular toileting 1 hour prior to the time of the fall reduce the risk of recurrence? Would a bed alarm alert the staff in time to assist the patient? These preventive strategies then would be developed into a fall prevention plan, individualized according to the needs of that particular patient.
- If it was an *anticipated physiological fall,* again meet with an interdisciplinary team to see if the possible cause of the fall may be rectified. For instance, if the fall was caused by fainting, examine the patient to identify the probable cause of the fainting, and develop a plan to prevent recurrence.

Finally, record the details of the fall in the *Falls Log Book* and develop a care plan by identifying fall prevention strategies to prevent recurrence. Fall prevention strategies will be described in the next section.

inability to go to the bathroom unassisted, use a bed alarm to alert staff that the patient is getting out of bed (See Appendix F for a list of manufactured alarms). Full-length side rails are dangerous because if the patient tries to climb over the top of the rail, he or she will have further to fall, and if the patient climbs out from the end of the bed, the fall is vertical. Thus, full-length side rails increase the chances of serious injury. Three-quarter length side rails should be used only to orient the patient to the side of the bed. Side rails are not restraints and should not be used to keep the patient in bed.

Ambulatory aids should aid patient mobility, yet they are often used inappropriately, thus increasing the risk of falling. Observe the patient using the walker: Many elderly *carry* the walker rather than use it as an assistive device. Make certain that the patient transfers safely from a chair to the walker or the wheelchair.

If the patient has nocturia, wake the patient during the night and assist the patient to the toilet. It may also be helpful to move patients at high risk of falling to rooms close to the nursing station, so that they may be observed more closely during the night.

Floors must not be highly polished because sunshine may create glare, causing temporary blindness in the elderly. Floors should be cleaned with a matte finish sealer.

Resident Teaching

Confused patients must be oriented constantly to their own [ ]ties, and the instruction that they must call the nurse if they wish [ ]t out of bed must be reinforced constantly. Instruction for use of [ ]ing aids, transferring techniques, and so forth must be repeated [ ]ently, and the patient's ability to use ambulatory aids should be [ ]essed often.

Increasing Staff Awareness

[ ]search has shown that many patients repeat a fall attemptin[ ] [ ]e activity that caused the first fall (Morse, Tylko, & Dixo[ ] [ ]Therefore, ensure that all staff are aware of the patients wh[ ]

Strategies for Preventing Falls

Strategies for preventing falls follow broad principles according to the type of fall (accidental, unanticipated physiological, and anticipated physiological) (see Chapter 1) and individualized plans to prevent a second fall, using information obtained from the fall assessment. Because patients fall in a variety of situations, and these falls are due to innumerable causes, there cannot be one routinized care plan to prevent falls. Although some prevention strategies are obvious and may be used with many patients, other patients present more of a challenge and demand creative and innovative solutions to ensure patient safety. Therefore, prevention strategies are not limited to those recommended here, and it is possible that important prevention strategies are still to be developed.

> Because residents fall in a variety of situations, and these falls are due to innumerable causes, there cannot be one routinized care plan to prevent falls.

In Table 5.1, the most frequently used fall prevention strategies identified in the literature are summarized (see Kilpatrick, Boehm, Smith, & Mudge, 1991; Ruckstuhl, Marchionda, Salmons, & Larrabee, 1991; Whedon & Shedd, 1989). In this table, these prevention strategies are sorted according to the type of fall that they might prevent.

Preventing *Anticipated Physiological Falls*

In this category, patients who score at risk of falling on the Morse Fall Scale are considered at risk of falling because they have physical conditions that contribute to that risk. The fall risk may be a general physical weakness, the effects of aging, or due to an illness or injury.

In the literature, there are several approaches to preventing anticipated physiological falls. The medical literature, not surprisingly, focuses on identifying the underlying conditions that contribute to the falling. More specifically, medical researchers' approaches to preventing patient falls are reflected as a relentless search for symptoms or diseases that result in the patient falls. Symptoms such as orthostatic hypotension (Campbell, Reinken, Allan, & Martinez, 1981; Davie, Blumenthal, & Robinson-Hewlens, 1981; Overstall, 1978; Tideiksaar & Kay, 1980), urinary frequency and urgency (Warshaw et al., 1982), problems with vision (Cohn & Lasley, 1985), mental confusion (Johnson, 1985), dehydration (Livesley & Atkinson, 1974), dizziness (Davie et al., 1981), balance and gait (Tinetti, Williams, & Mayewski, 1986; Wolfson, Whipple, Amerman, Kaplan, & Kleinberg, 1985), or "drop attacks" (Brocklehurst, Exton-Smith, & Barber, 1978; Lipsitz, 1983) have been associated with falling. Other researchers have investigated specific diseases that contribute to patient falls, such as Alzheimer's disease (Morris, Rubin, Morris, & Mandel, 1987), Parkinson's disease (Grant & Hamilton, 1987), CVAs (Grant & Hamilton, 1987), the presence of multiple illnesses (Tinetti et al., 1986), or advancing age (Warshaw et al., 1982).

Assessment forms created by physician investigators consist of long checklists searching for the physiological cause of the fall [e.g., The Gait Abnormality Rating Scale (Wolfson, Whipple, Amerman, & Tobin, 1990); Appendix 1 from the Physical Examination Guidelines (Tideiksaar, 1989); and the Fall Risk Assessment Form (Tideiksaar, 1984)]. Thus, should the high score be illness related, it is important to draw the physician's attention to a patient who has a high fall score—in particular, if the fall has not yet occurred.

Polypharmacy is frequently a problem with elderly patients and those with more than one diagnosis, and some researchers have focused their interventions on this area. Pharmacists should be consulted to see if the high fall score risk possibly could be attributed in part to drug interactions. Certain classes of drugs have been correlated with patients who fall. For instance, diuretics, sedatives, analgesics, hypnotics, and antihypertensives all have been associated with patient falls.

Engineers have focused their prevention efforts on ways to adapt the environment to prevent falls, or, if a fall occurs, they have modified the environment to reduce the chance of injury. These researchers have focused on optimal lighting, the position of handrails, bed designs, and so forth. Because fall-prone patients have a weak impaired gait, often due to a loss of balance, check that the environment is arranged for maximal safety. Handrails (31 inches from fl with a round grip) should be installed in the patient's room bet the bed and the bathroom. If this is not possible, create a path bathroom with sturdy, nonskid, waist-high furniture for the pat use as support when moving unassisted to the bathroom. Che appropriate handrails are installed in the bathroom, and h bathroom call bell within easy reach of the toilet. Again, nig must be installed, so that the patient will be oriented quickly her surroundings when waking at night and so that he or she quickly to the bathroom.

Nursing research, on the other hand, has focused on ventions that will reduce the patient's risk of falling. explored such things as observing and assisting the patient, toileting, exercising, and teaching the patient. Nursing research has noted that it is important that those who score high on the scale should be identified. Then, any staff member will be able to recognize fall-prone patients immediately and provide assistance if necessary. So these high-risk patients by placing a colored s doors; beside their beds; on their walkers, can their charts; and beside their call bells.

Most of the falls occ patient is getting ou must be kept in the except when care tered to the patie

Studies have shown that most of the falls is getting out of bed. As a matter of policy kept in the low position, except when care the patient. If the patient is confused and

have fallen, the time of the occurrence, and the patient activity at the time of the fall so that a second fall may be prevented. For example, if a patient fell while going to the bathroom at 3 a.m., staff should routinely wake the patient and assist him or her to the toilet at 2 a.m. Do not leave the patient unattended on the commode because patients are often at risk of falling after a bowel movement.

Regularly Monitor the Patient's Fall Score

Observe for particular times throughout the day when the score increases. For example, the score may increase in the afternoons because the patient is tired and the fatigue is noticeable in changes in gait. Provide extra precautionary measures at these times.

Attempt to Decrease Fall Score by Consulting With the Interdisciplinary Committee

If, for example, the patient's gait is impaired or weak, a physical therapist should be consulted to see if a program of exercise will increase muscular strength and improve gait. If the patient is on multiple medications, ask the pharmacist to check for drug interactions and, if possible, have the number of medications reduced.

Unfortunately, all fall prevention strategies cannot be listed. Sometimes, identifying the appropriate fall prevention strategy requires creativity and innovation from the nurse. For example, an elderly patient was restless and wandering, and the staff were reluctant to restrain him. When the patient's son offered to bring in the patient's own arm chair, the staff agreed to try it. The change was remarkable—the patient immediately was settled and content in his chair, and the wandering behavior ceased.

Another strategy was less successful. A patient was constantly trying to get out of bed, and the staff were concerned that the patient would fall from the bed. The staff decided to reduce the patient's risk and removed the patient's bed, leaving only a mattress on the floor. The patient continued to be restless; he stood up and tripped over the mattress.

Multiple Fallers

Patients who fall are likely to fall again. Repeated falls account for a large percentage of the total falls in an institution—from approximately 20% in an acute care hospital (Morse, Prowse, Morrow, & Federspeil, 1985) to 50% in a nursing home population (Wright, Aizenstein, Vogler, Rowe, & Miller, 1990), and in one study, multiple fallers accounted for as much as 70% of all falls (Sehested & Severin-Nielsen, 1977). Although studies have shown that a patient is most likely to fall during the first week of hospitalization (when 3 out of every 10 elderly patients fall) (Catchen, 1983), the patient's likelihood of repeating a fall is associated with length of stay, and the longer a patient remains in hospital, the greater the likelihood that a fall will be repeated. Furthermore, it has been shown that an increase in repeated falls is due to increasing debility, and that falls tend to cluster around the time of death (Gryfe, Amies, & Ashley, 1977).

===

In 55% of the cases, the first and second fall occurred in similar circumstances, often at the same time of day.

===

Monitoring Individuals Who Fall: Identifying Patterns

Repeated falls are not a random event. Examination of the circumstances and time of the repeated fall revealed that in 55% of the cases, the first and second fall occurred in similar circumstances (i.e., the patient was repeating the same activity), often at approximately the same time of day (Morse, Tylko, & Dixon, 1985). These patterns of falling become clear when examining data from a patient's chart:

Fall #1:   2.35 p.m.   Patient fell while climbing out of bed unassisted.
Fall #2:   3.10 a.m.   Patient found on floor beside bed. Disoriented.

Fall #3: 2.45 p.m. Patient climbed out of bed unassisted.
Slipped on urine.

Fall #4: 1.50 p.m. Patient went to bathroom unassisted.
Patient fell from commode.

From the above, it is clear that the nursing interventions should be to ensure that the patient empties his or her bladder prior to a nap and that he or she is woken from the nap—and also at about 2 a.m.—for toileting. Therefore, when a patient falls, it is important to make the staff aware of the fall and the time and circumstances of the fall to prevent recurrence.

A recording system for highlighting the times and circumstances of falls is essential. Writing the details in the patient's chart is inadequate because the entry quickly becomes "archived" and lost between entries. Thus, in addition to reporting the fall in the patient's chart, it is recommended that a *Fall Log Book* be kept in the nursing station. A fall log book is a notebook in which every fall is recorded—who, where, when, and what, plus the nursing recommendations for prevention of a second fall. Each patient who falls should have a separate page, so that all falls for the same patient are recorded on the same list. Nurses may then look at the entries and quickly discern circumstances that place each patient at risk of a fall, which strategies for prevention have been tried, which strategies have worked to prevent the fall, and which strategies have not worked.

> Keep a *Fall Log Book* in each unit.

Developing a Care Plan for Fall Prevention

To prevent an anticipated fall (or the second unanticipated physiological fall), it is recommended that the identified fall prevention strategies be incorporated onto the patient's care plan. It is inadequate simply to write: "Fall precautions." The interventions for each patient should be noted specifically. Ensure that the times that the patient is most at risk—times the patient voids or is restless at night—are listed.

Providing Adequate Walking Aids

In most institutions, essential departments close over weekends and holidays. This means that patients admitted during these times must wait—sometimes several days—until issued with an appropriate walking frame, crutches, or cane. Such delays place the patient at high risk of falling, and such institutional policies contribute to the high rate of falling in patients soon after admission.

Special Equipment

Very elderly patients, who cannot bear weight or stand without assistance and yet are very restless, are often frail and confused. If left unattended in bed, they tend to move about the bed and may even try to exit the bed through the side rails. When sitting in a gerichair, they tend to slip under the tray. Beanbag chairs (hospital quality) are the ideal solution for these patients. These chairs provide the patient with adequate back support and allow freedom of movement, but the sides of the beanbag provide enough support to prevent the patient from crawling out. However, it is important not to leave these patients unattended: They require careful monitoring.

Using Side Rails: *Not* a Fall Prevention Strategy

Many authors have listed "keeping the side rails up" as a fall prevention strategy (e.g., see Berryman, Gaskin, Jones, Tolley, & MacMullen, 1989). It is important to note that side rails will not keep a patient in bed. Any patient who is restless should have his or her side rails up, but these side rails will not prevent a patient from climbing out of bed. At best, side rails do two things: (a) They may serve as a reminder to the patients that they are not sleeping in a double bed and can locate the edge of the mattress;

> Side rails are ineffective as a strategy to keep a patient in bed and increase the risk of injury to the patient.

and (b) they provide a handhold so that patients can pull themselves up to a sitting position. Side rails *will not keep a patient in bed* and even increase the risk of injury should a patient decide to climb out of bed. With the side rails up, the patient who decides to get out of bed must then climb over the top of the rail (and therefore have a greater distance to fall to the floor), try to leave the bed by going over the foot of the bed (and this is a "vertical cliff," increasing the likelihood of falling), or go through the side rail and risk strangulation. Side rails, therefore, are ineffective as a strategy to keep a patient in bed and increase the risk of injury to the patient. If side rails are used with a confused and restless patient, then the patient should be monitored constantly.

Assessment for Using a Bed Alarm

Alarms alert the nurses only when a patient begins to get out of the bed. Because nurses may be assisting another patient in another part of the unit, it may be several minutes before a nurse can assist the patient when an alarm sounds. Staff must therefore expect that the patient will get out of bed and stand. Therefore, the patient must have a safe route to get out of the bed. *Full-length side rails must never be used* because they force the patient to climb over the top of the rail or to climb over the foot of the bed. Both of these actions *increase* the risk of falling and injury. Ideally, three-quarter-length side rails should be used. Because the patient will have to slide down the bed to exit, this will delay the exit, giving the nurse more time to get to the bedside. It provides the safest way for the patient to slide out of bed feet first, and the side rail provides a handhold and will help support the patient.

> Bed alarms are most useful when a patient has a normal or weak gait, is confused, and attempts to get out of bed at night and wander.

Thus, bed alarm systems that alert staff when a patient is attempting to get out of bed are helpful in the following instances:

1. The patient can bear weight, so that as the patient exits the bed, he or she can stand beside the bed, holding on to the side rail until help arrives.
2. The patient is confused and forgets to use the call bell to ask for assistance when getting out of bed. The patient overestimates his or her own abilities and thinks that he or she can go to the bathroom without assistance.
3. The patient does not have an impaired gait. Because it may take many seconds for a staff member to reach the patient, the patient may attempt to walk before the nurse reaches the bedside. Therefore, if the patient has an impaired gait, he or she is at risk of falling before assistance arrives.

Thus, bed alarms are most useful when a patient has a normal or weak gait, is confused, and attempts to get out of bed at night and wander.

The Use of Mechanical Restraints

In hospitals, restraints are used for five reasons: to protect patients from self-injurious behaviors (such as in psychiatric units) or from interfering with equipment or treatments (such as IV tubing, catheters, or monitors); to prevent an elderly, confused person from wandering away from the unit or an elderly frail person from falling; or finally, Strumpf, Evans, and Schwartz (1990) noted that they may be used as a punitive measure or to force patient compliance.

> Patients who were restrained showed an increased occurrence of fall-related injuries.

Paradoxically, the use of a mechanical restraint to prevent a serious injury may actually increase risk to the patient. There is no evidence that the use of restraints prevents patient accidents ("Restraints," 1980). Restraints have been directly attributed to such accidents as hanging or asphyxiation because of the patient's head being caught in the side rail (David, 1987). Patients also have pulled furniture on top of themselves or have become tangled in the restraint straps ("Restraints," 1980). The use of restraints makes patients passive and dependent, and Wendkos (1980) reports that one patient became so distressed at being "tied up" that the patient died a sudden death. Of concern, there is dubious value in the use of mechanical restraints to prevent a patient from falling. The use of mechanical restraints may contribute to cognitive impairment (Burton, German, Rovner, & Brant, 1992); patients who were restrained showed an increased occurrence of fall-related injuries compared with nonrestrained patients (Tinetti, Liu, & Ginter, 1992); and, following the removal of restraints, the rate of nonserious falls increased, but serious falls did not increase (Ejaz, Jones, & Rose, 1994). When comparing the care provided to patients who were restrained and then had their restraints removed, Morse and McHutchion (1991) found that whereas the number of nurse contacts with nonrestrained patients was higher than that for restrained patients, the actual contact time for providing care decreased.

The federal and state regulations for the use of mechanical and chemical restraints are changing rapidly, and if restraints are used within an institution, care must be taken to ensure that the institution is in compliance with all regulations. All alternatives to a restraint must be explored first. For instance, it may be feasible to find volunteers to sit with the patient for a part of the day, thus rendering restraints unnecessary for long periods of time. Once the decision to use mechanical restraints has been made, the patient's guardian must be consulted because the guardian has the right of refusal.

A mechanical restraint is defined as any manual method of mechanical device, material, or equipment attached or adjacent to the patient's body that the patient cannot remove easily, and which restricts freedom of movement. A chemical restraint is a psychopharmaceutical drug that is not required to treat medical symptoms but is used for behavioral management of the patient. Note that restrictive devices that act as a reminder to the patient are *not* restraints. These include Velcro belts to prevent the patient from falling from a wheelchair but that the patient may remove him- or herself. These devices are dangerous *if* the staff rely on them as if they were restraints—and the patient removes them, "escapes," stands, and then falls.

A physician's order is required for the application of a mechanical restraint, and the reason for its application must be charted. Nursing care must include special surveillance and protective measures to prevent injury caused by the use of these devices. Such measures include the following:

- Observing the patient closely, in particular for the first 24 hours
- Applying the restraint correctly, so that the patient's circulation, sensation, and respirations are not impaired; loosen restraints every 2 hours so that the patient can cough, breathe deeply, and exercise; and monitor vital signs
- Checking the circulation of the extremities every 15 minutes for as long as the restraint is applied
- Providing a change of positions and range of motion for not less than 10 minutes every 2 hours
- Toileting the patient every 2 hours

On the nurse's care plan, document the type of restraint, the reason for its application, the physician's order, the discussion with the patient and the family, and the patient's reaction. Initiate a behavior monitoring sheet. Document the patient reaction to the restraint. Document the frequency with which the restraint was checked, removed, and reassessed to ensure comfort, circulation, movement, and sensation. Reassess periodically the need for the continued use of the restraint.

Preventing *Unanticipated Physiological Falls*

As described earlier, the goal for *unanticipated physiological falls* is to prevent subsequent falls or prevent the patient from injury should a second fall occur. Recognize that the possibility of falls occurs with certain conditions and circumstances, such as drug interactions and illnesses. For example, nurses learn to watch and automatically assist patients who are likely to fall when they are getting out of bed for the first time after an illness. Resident/patient teaching is an important component of preventing the recurrence of the unanticipated fall: Patients with epilepsy must be taught how to recognize an aura, and patients

Resident/patient teaching is an important component of preventing the recurrence of the unanticipated fall.

with orthostatic hypotension should be taught how to get up slowly when lying in bed and to seek assistance when getting up.

When a second unanticipated fall is unavoidable, protective devices will help to prevent the patient from injury when a second fall occurs. Patients with epilepsy may be provided with helmets to prevent a head injury should a seizure occur, and hip pads may prevent the elderly person prone to falls from receiving a serious hip injury.

Preventing *Accidental Falls*

Accidental falls occur when the patient slips or trips over something in the environment, rather than being caused by some factor that may be attributed to the illness or injury. Accidental falls are prevented by ensuring a safe environment and orienting the patient to that environment.

Ensuring a Safe Environment

A detailed description of ensuring a safe environment has been presented in Chapter 2, so only the main points will be summarized here. Although it is obvious to note that long-term care equipment must be well maintained, nurses often tolerate poorly maintained equipment. For example, nurses may hesitate to send a wheelchair for repair because they do not have a replacement to use while the faulty one is being repaired. Thus, a program of regular, systematic maintenance checks should be established. Wheelchairs must be checked to ensure that the brakes hold and that the foot pedals lift aside easily. Beds are checked to ensure that the brakes hold, even if a patient leans against the bed, and that the side rails do not give way when leaned on. Step stools used to climb in and out of bed are dangerous and should be used only with nursing assistance, if at all. If used, make certain that the stool is stable and has a nonskid base. Check that each leg has a rubber, nonskid foot.

Equipment that patients use to assist with walking must be checked. If a walker has wheels, ensure that the axles of these wheels are clean and oiled so that they move freely and do not stick. Similarly, the wheels on any furniture or equipment that the patient uses as a walking aid must move freely. The low-high adjustment of IV poles should be easily moveable because if they are stiff and difficult to lower, patients, when walking about the unit, may catch these poles on the tops of doorways or on overhead rails (or patients may try to walk looking up to see if it will catch) and lose their balance.

Although the impervious nature of the floor covering is important for hygienic reasons, it is also a hazard should anything be spilled on the floor and not cleaned immediately. To prevent slips, any spilled urine or water must be wiped up immediately and the floors kept clean and dry. The floors should be cleaned with a matte finish floor sealer. If the floor is carpeted, the flooring should be free of any kinks, loose edges, threads, or tears that may trip the patient. Loose rugs should not be used. The flooring should be even and should not contain any wooden strips, steps, or stairs.

Ensure that there are adequate railings and that these railings are in the areas most needed by the patients. They should be in the patients' rooms, providing a secure handhold between the bed and the bathroom. Call bells should be in easy reach, especially in the bathroom.

Accidental falls are prevented by ensuring a safe environment and orienting the resident to that environment.

Orienting the Patient to the Environment

Because a greater proportion of falls occurs during the first week of hospitalization, orienting the patient to the new environment is important. Furthermore, if the patient is confused, this orientation should be an ongoing process. The use of night lights will assist the elderly patient in finding his or her way to the bathroom at night. Patients also must be shown how to use the call bell, and they should be instructed to use it when requiring assistance (rather than calling or shouting for the nurse). Newly admitted patients should be checked routinely at regular intervals during the night until their habits are known to the staff and the patient is familiar with his or her new surroundings.

Staff Awareness

The success of the program is dependent on building and maintaining continual awareness of the fall risk of certain high-risk patients and of fall prevention strategies. Labeling the charts of certain high-risk patients with a sticker denoting their high-risk status is important. However, most important is the support that staff receive from administration. If staff notify the supervisor that they have a "difficult" patient at high risk for falls and require extra staff or a volunteer to sit with the patient, and if such relief is not provided, then staff will become discouraged and feel that they have few options in reducing fall risk. Preventing a fall will appear an impossible task.

6

Evaluating the Effectiveness
of a Program

The long-term success of a fall prevention program is dependent on
the continuous effort of the caregivers and the commitment of staff
and administration for fall prevention. Caregivers must be constantly
aware of each patient's fall risk and always vigilant, ready to protect
the patient from falling.

Why Do We Evaluate Fall Prevention Programs?

Earlier, it was mentioned that a fall that was circumvented successfully frequently went unnoticed. Just like a near-miss car accident,
a prevented fall has no cost savings per se because the damaging event
did not occur. If a fall does occur, the patient may or may not be
injured, and the accident is considered an "incident" only *if* the patient

is injured. Thus, with a *prevented* fall, because the fall did not occur, the question of what kind of injury was prevented becomes only a hypothetical question. Nevertheless, evaluation of a fall prevention program serves three important functions. First, it enables estimation of the cost of falls to the health care system and the institution and, from that, the cost savings from a fall prevention program. Second, the evaluation enables the identification of the pattern of falls in an institution and the targeting of areas that are of high risk. Finally, it provides important feedback to staff and the institution that the fall program is indeed working to reduce falls.

Evaluation of a fall prevention program

• Enables estimation of the cost of falls to the health care system
• Identifies patterns of falls within an institution
• Provides a system of monitoring the effectiveness of the fall prevention program

First, the overall economic cost can be estimated for patient falls and applied in principle to the reduction in fall rate. Nationally, the cost per annum for patient falls has been estimated at billions of dollars (Baker & Harvey, 1985). Whereas the cost to a single institution of a fall resulting in an injury is variable (depending on the severity of the injury and so forth), the dollar cost and the cost in human suffering and subsequent decrease in the quality of life is considerable.

Once the dollar costs have been identified, then the *reductions* in the number of falls following the implementation of the fall prevention programs may be considered as savings. Note, however, that we have not attempted to place a dollar cost on the human pain and suffering caused by the fall nor on the legal ramifications of a fall, should a lawsuit follow.

The second important function of the evaluation of the programs is derived from the accumulation of statistics and descriptive information about individual patients who fall. From these data, patterns of falls within an institution may be developed. For instance, areas in which different patients fall often can be identified as high risk for accidental falls, and the factors that may be contributing to the fall can be identified and corrected. For example, if several patients fall in front of the nurses' station, examine the area carefully. One may notice, for instance, that there is a large space of more than 15 feet that patients must cross and in which there are no handholds or railings. Placing a table in this space that patients can use as a support or at which they can sit and rest will reduce the falls in this area.

On the other hand, if one patient falls repeatedly, commonalities about the time, place, and circumstances of the fall may be identified, and the circumstances surrounding the future fall event predicted and prevented. Such preventive measures cannot be implemented without an evaluation program consisting of careful monitoring and feedback provided to the staff. In this way, the evaluation of the fall prevention program becomes a matter of comparing fall and injury rates after the implementation of the program with those before the program and noting/counting the near misses as successful interventions.

Third, the compilation and monitoring of patient falls and injuries provide a system of monitoring the effectiveness of the fall prevention program. As mentioned previously, effective monitoring involves regular communication to all staff. It also involves regular comparisons, both monthly and annually, for selected patient populations and all units.

Evaluating Successful Interventions

The irony of fall prevention programs is that if a fall is *prevented,* then it is as though *it did not happen.* Whereas a fall may cost many thousands of dollars, there may be no cost savings with a prevented fall because the fall did not actually occur.

The success of particular interventions is therefore difficult to assess. Following an environmental inspection of a unit, the repair of wheelchairs and other equipment, the removal of shiny floor polish, and so forth, the only indicator of "success" will be the general reduction of accidental falls. If new handrails were installed, observing the use of these rails is not necessarily an indication that the rails have actually prevented a fall. Occasionally, it is easier to identify an intervention that has averted a fall. This may be most evident with patients who have fallen repeatedly while attempting to do the same thing. For instance, if a patient has fallen on several occasions when going to the bathroom about 3 a.m., and the intervention identified was to wake the patient at 2 a.m. for toileting, and the patient subsequently did not attempt to get out of bed at 3 a.m., and had not fallen during a reasonable period of time, the staff may consider this intervention "successful." However, for continued success, all staff, including relief staff, must be aware of this patient's special needs.

Staff Monitoring

Because of the relatively weak and serendipitous association between fall prevention strategies and the actual prevention of a fall, it is imperative that there be active communication of fall prevention strategies between staff. Methods of monitoring fall-prone patients and prevention strategies must be incorporated into the patient's care plan and reinforced on each change of shift report.

> Incorporate fall prevention strategies into the patient's care plan and reinforce these at each change of shift report.

The significance of reporting all falls on the incident report form —whether or not an injury occurs—must be stressed to staff. While such reporting may result initially in an increase in the number of falls (at a time when a new prevention program has been introduced), these falls are important. Recall that if a patient is not injured in a fall, that may be considered a lucky event. And because the patient may fall again doing the same thing, reporting the fall will bring the risk of a subsequent fall to everyone's attention and permit preventive strategies to be identified and put into place.

Institutional Tracking

Because hospitals organize patients' units by diagnosis, patients' risk of falling varies from unit to unit. Thus, patients' fall scores vary from unit to unit. In surgical units, patients tend to be younger, are admitted with a normal gait, and then, following surgery, develop a weak gait and have an IV. In the surgical units, the scores tend to be lower than those for a cardiac medical unit or a psychogeriatric unit. Surgical units tend to show a large range of variability over the course of the average 10-day hospital stay and also throughout a 24-hour day. On the other hand, in a unit with older patients, such as a psychogeriatric unit with Alzheimer's patients, all patients in the unit will have a higher fall score because of an impaired gait, impaired mental status, a history of falling, and use of walking aids. Patients on this unit will tend to show a more stable fall score with less variation over a 24-hour period and less variation from day to day. The risk of patients falling in the surgical unit is much less than the risk of falling in the psychogeriatric unit. Thus, it is important that institutional tracking for the number of falls, monthly or annually, be reported by unit as well as by the institution as a whole. Regular calculation of the fall rate is important to identify areas or units in the institution that require special attention for fall prevention and thus provide extra staff to assist with residents or with modifications to the environment.

Increase in the reporting of falls by staff occurs with the implementation of a fall prevention program rather than an actual increase in the number of falls.

Monthly calculations of the fall rate and reporting of these fall rates to all staff serve as a reminder to staff about the importance of prevention. But do not forget that the implementation of a fall prevention program often results in an increase in the *reporting of falls* by staff rather than an increase in the number of falls that actually occur. The increased reporting, just as the prevention program is initiated, probably represents a more accurate fall rate (with staff underreporting previously) rather than an actual increase in the number of falls. It is recommended that the *injury rate* also be calculated because this may be a more reliable indicator of the effectiveness of the program. If the injury rate has decreased over a period of several months, then it is probable that the fall prevention program is working successfully to reduce the number of falls. Keep in mind, however, that the fall rate of one unit may fluctuate over a short period of time and appear unstable. The presence of one person who continues to fall repeatedly despite the efforts of staff to intervene may result in dramatic, short-term increases in the fall rates of one particular unit.

Providing Feedback to Staff

Providing regular feedback to staff reminds staff of the importance of fall prevention and provides satisfaction in the knowledge that their efforts are indeed working. The statistics should be placed in each unit on a form. An example of a reporting form is shown in Figure 6.1.

Institutional Monitoring

The compilation of fall statistics by the institution should ideally include the following information: fall rate, injury rate, and Morse fall score. Information about the type of fall (anticipated or unanticipated physiological, or accidental) as well as patient demographics also may be useful to the institution for research purposes.

The Last Word

Several things are critical for the successful implementation of a fall prevention program, and they are worth repeating:

- If a patient falls, it is a failed strategy; not a nurse's "fault." Exploring why a patient fell, rather than who "let" the patient fall, is the first step in developing a fall prevention program.
- Preventing falls is the responsibility of the total institution, not just the nursing staff. Housekeeping, medical staff—and even engineering and

FALL PREVENTION REPORT

Statistics for (date) _____   Unit _____

Number of falls _____   Number of injuries _____

Level of Injury

Minor _____   Moderate _____   Serious _____

Fall Rate _____   Injury Rate _____

Repeated falls

	Patients	Room/Bed #	Number of falls
1.	_____	_____	_____
2.	_____	_____	_____
3.	_____	_____	_____
4.	_____	_____	_____
5.	_____	_____	_____
6.	_____	_____	_____

Rating

Unit   Institution

Figure 6.1. Example of an Institutional Report Form

the physical plant—have responsibility and can make contributions to patient safety.

- The Morse Fall Scale does not prevent falls—it only identifies those patients at risk of falling. It is the identification and implementation of fall prevention strategies that prevent patient falls.

- A patient who experiences an unanticipated physiological fall is likely to fall again, doing the same thing, and probably at the same time of day.

Appendix A

Alternative Assessment Scales

The available scales to identify the fall-prone patient and to differentiate between the types of scales or instruments available are reviewed in this appendix. Note that the variables included in the instruments to detect patients likely to fall or to identify the factors that may contribute to a patient falling reflect the disciplinary bias of the researcher. For example, physicians have tended to look for symptoms or clusters of symptoms that occur in patients who are likely to fall; pharmacists look for patterns of drug interactions or side effects of drugs that may contribute to a patient fall; physical therapists examine gait and balance; whereas nurses have tended to focus on patient behaviors that may contribute to a fall, such as patterns of voiding or urinary urgency, failure to use the call bell or to ask for assistance when getting out of bed, or staffing levels or activities (such as time of staff report) that are ongoing when the fall occurs. These perspectives have profound implications for the management of or the approach to a fall prevention program. For example, the medical approach to patient falls (i.e., considering the fall as a *symptom* of a disease) implies that the patient must fall—exhibit the symptom—before the cause of the fall is investigated. Thus, the focus must be on the *prevention of a repeated fall.*

Risk Assessment Forms

There are 12 forms available that predict the patient's risk of falling, and these are listed in Table A.1. When reviewing these forms, it is wise to check on the derivation of the form. Look for information

Table A.1 Comparison of Variables in Fall-Assessment Forms

Variable	Barbieri (1983)	Berryman et al. (1989)	Fife et al. (1984)	Hendrich (1988)	Innes & Turman (1983)	Kallmann et al. (1992)	Llewellyn et al. (1988)	Morse et al. (1989)	Rainville (1984)	Spellbring et al. (1988)	Tack et al. (1987)	Young et al. (1989)
Age	—	X	X	X	—	X	X	—	X	X	X	—
Sex	—	—	X	X	—	—	—	—	X	—	—	X
History of falling	X	X	X	—	—	X	X	X	—	X	—	—
Secondary diagnosis	X	—	—	—	—	—	—	X	—	X	—	—
Condition												
Weakness	X	—	X	X	?	—	—	—	—	—	—	X
Dizzyness	X	—	X	—	—	X	—	—	—	X	?	X
Gait	X	X	—	?	—	—	X	X	—	X	—	X
Incontinence/Urgency	X	—	—	X	?	—	—	—	—	X	—	—
Sensory deficit												
Visual	X	X	X	—	X	X	—	—	—	X	X	X
Auditory	X	—	X	—	—	—	—	—	—	X	X	X
Communication	—	—	—	—	X	—	?	—	—	X	X	X
Mental status	—	—	X	X	X	X	X	X	X	X	X	X
Attitude/depression	X	—	—	—	X	—	—	—	—	X	—	X
Ambulatory aids	—	—	X	—	—	—	—	X	—	—	X	X
Restraints	—	—	X	—	—	—	—	—	—	—	X	X
Footwear	X	—	—	—	X	—	—	—	—	X	—	X

	Patient's knowledge	Elimination	Post-op	Elevated temperature	Post-op	Elimination	Length of stay	IV therapy	Length of stay	Orthostatic hypotension	Physical limitations	Escape restraints
Medications												
Diuretics	X	X	X	X	X	X	—	—	—	X	X	X
Analgesics	X	—	X	X	—	—	—	—	—	X	X	X
Hypnotics/tranquilizers	X	X	X	X	X	X	—	—	—	X	X	X
Laxatives/cathartics	—	—	X	X	X	X	—	—	—	X	X	X
Environment	—	—	—	—	X	—	—	—	—	—	—	—
Other		Length of stay Confined to a chair Blood pressure				Confined to a chair Increase in blood pressure						
Comments	Care plan			Form also serves as fall report	Care plan		Prescriptive care plan			Includes prevention	Includes fall report	Form identifies patients at risk and care plans

81

about the methods of scale construction, reliability and validity information, and information regarding posttesting of the instrument. Table 1.2 displays a comparison of the checklist for forms for the prevention of patient falls. The most comprehensive list is by Spellbring, Gannon, Kleckner, and Conway (1988). However, although these checklists may be of some use as a reminder to ensure that all steps have been taken in prevention, they are of little use to the bedside nurse in his or her day-to-day efforts to prevent falls.

Table A.2 Comparison of Intervention Checklists for the Prevention of Patient Falls

Intervention	Fife et al. (1984)	Innes & Turman (1983)	Llewellyn et al. (1988)	Rainville (1984)	Spellbring et al. (1988)	Tack et al. (1987)
Identify potential to fall	—	—	—	—	X	—
Orient to environment	—	—	—	—	X	—
Night light	—	—	—	X	X	X
Evaluate medications	X	X	X	—	X	—
Furniture	—	X	X	X	X	—
Assist to void	—	—	X	—	X	—
Bedlow, locked	—	—	—	X	X	—
Side rails	X	X	X	X	X	—
Restraints/safety belt	X	X	X	—	X	X
Call bell	—	—	—	X	X	—
Walking aides	X	—	—	—	X	—
Footwear	—	X	X	—	X	X
Check patient	—	X	X	—	X	X
Reinforce risk with patient	—	X	—	X	X	X
Involve family	—	X	—	X	X	X

Appendix B

Development of the Morse Fall Scale

The procedure for developing the *Morse Fall Scale* was, briefly, (a) establishing a database from 100 patients who fell and 100 randomly selected patients who had not fallen; (b) identifying the significant variables that differentiate the fallers from the nonfallers; (c) obtaining scale weights for each item; (d) using the weights from these significant variables to calculate item values and to determine the scale score that classifies patients at risk of falling; (e) computer testing the scale on a simulated patient population (obtained from the original database); (f) estimating the reliability; and (g) establishing validity by randomly splitting the data set, repeating Steps 2 through 4 on one half of the data, and, using discriminant analysis, testing the subsequently derived scale variables on the other half of the data.[1]

1. The Establishment of a Database

The examination of 100 patients who fell and 100 controls (i.e., randomly selected patients who had not fallen) provided a database for the development of the scale. A fall was defined as an event in which the patient came to rest on the floor (see Morris & Isaacs, 1980). This definition includes patients slipping from the chair to the floor and patients found lying on the floor and listed as fallen (i.e., falls in which a bystander caught the patient, and, although the impact of the fall was prevented, the patient was lowered onto the floor). Variables collected included physiological and environmental variables from both groups, and, for the fall group, information pertaining to the circumstances of the fall. Data were obtained from the patients' charts and by examining the patient and inspecting the environment. Comparisons were made using the chi-square test and the Kolmogorov-Smirnov two-sample test.

Comparison of patients who had fallen with the control group showed that the following variables were not significant: the sex of the patient, primary diagnosis, orthostatic hypotension, temperature, hemoglobin, presence of diarrhea or vomiting, method of voiding, visual impairments, or hearing deficits. The control group was significantly younger than the fall group, and 58% of the patients that fell were between 65 and 89 years of age. Of significance, the fall group was hospitalized longer, $p = .02$; had fallen before, $p < .0005$; had more than one diagnosis, $p < .0005$; were confused, $p < .0005$; had nocturia with urgency, $p = .02$; had abnormal skin turgor, $p = .05$; had an IV, $p < .0005$; used oxygen, $p = .05$; and were less likely to experience pain that interfered with movement, $p = .01$. The fall group was also more likely to have an abnormal gait, $p < .0005$, and to require nursing assistance or crutches, a cane, or a walker when ambulating, $p < .0005$ (Morse et al., 1987). A complete listing of variables included in this analysis is shown in Table B.1.

2. Identifying Significant Variables

Discriminant analysis was used to classify individuals according to the criterion variable (i.e., whether or not the patient had fallen). The discriminant classification is based on an index derived from scores obtained from a set of discriminant variables. Six variables met the significant criterion of $F > .001$ as minimum tolerance level. These were history of falling (i.e., a previous fall), presence of a secondary diagnosis, use of intravenous therapy, type of gait (i.e., normal, weak, or impaired), the type and use of ambulatory aids, and mental status (see Note 1).

The variables were defined as follows:

Table B.1 Comparison of Patients Who Fell With Randomized Controls:
Significant and Nonsignificant Variables

Significant Variables	p	Nonsignificant Variables
Age	.000	Sex
Length of hospitalization	.002	
History of falling	.000	
Secondary diagnosis	.000	Primary diagnosis
Mental status	.000	Height
Skin turgor	.002	Weight
Respirator: Use of O$_2$	.05	Diarrhea
Pulse rate	.02	Vomiting
Pain	.01	Bowel sounds
Nocturia with urgency	.05	Hemoglobin
IV therapy	.000	Orthostatic hypotension
Vision: use of lens	.04	
Gait	.000	
Walking aids	.000	
Side rails	.002	

History of Falling. This was coded as 1 if a previous fall was
recorded during the present hospital admission, or if there was an
immediate history of physiological falls, such as from seizures or an
impaired gait, prior to admission.

Secondary Diagnosis. This was coded as 1 if more than one medical diagnosis was listed on the patient's chart.

Ambulatory Aids. This was coded as 0 if the patient walked without a walking aid (even if assisted by a nurse) or was on bed rest. If
the patient used crutches, a cane, or a walker, this was coded as 1, or
as 2 if the patient ambulated clutching onto the furniture for support.

Intravenous Therapy. This was coded as 1 if the patient had an
intravenous apparatus or a heparin lock inserted.

Gait. The characteristics of the three types of gait were evident regardless of the type of physical disability. A normal gait is characterized by the patient walking with head erect, arms swinging freely at the side and striding unhesitantly, and was coded as 0.

With a *weak gait* (coded as 1), the patient is stooped but is able to lift his or her head while walking. Support from furniture is sought, but this is a featherweight touch, almost for reassurance. Steps are short and the patient may shuffle.

With an *impaired gait* (coded as 2), the patient may have difficulty rising from the chair, attempts to rise by pushing on the arms of the chair and/or by bouncing. The patient's head is down, and, because the balance is poor, the patient grasps onto the furniture, a support person, or a walking aid for support and cannot walk without this assistance. The steps are short and the patient shuffles.

If the patient was in a wheelchair, the patient was scored according to the gait he or she used when transferring from the wheelchair to the bed.

Mental Status. In this study, mental status was measured by checking the patient's own self-assessment of ambulatory ability. The patient was asked if he or she was able to go to the bathroom alone, if he or she needed assistance, or if he or she was permitted up. If the patient's assessment was consistent with the ambulatory orders on the Kardex®, the patient was rated as normal and coded 0. If the patient's response was not consistent with these orders, or if the patient's assessment was unrealistic, then the patient was considered to overestimate his or her own abilities and to be forgetful of limitations, and thus coded as 1.

In this study, the dependent variable was dichotomous (i.e., each subject could be classified as either a faller or a control). Therefore, if a patient was randomly classified in either the fall group or the control group, there was a 50% probability of a correct classification.

When performing discriminant analysis, four groups are obtained, as follows:

	Actual Group	
Predicted Group	Fall	Control
Fall	Falls correct (True positive)	Controls incorrect (False positive)
Control	Falls incorrect (False negative)	Controls correct (True negative)

In the study, the discriminant solution, using the six significant variables, correctly classified 78% of the fall group and 83% of the control group (total correct: 80.5%). This result is significantly greater than the 50% that would be expected to occur by chance. Results were as follows:

	Actual Group	
Predicted Group	Fall	Control
Fall (n = 100)	78 (39%)	17 (8.5%)
Control (n = 100)	22 (11%)	83 (41.5%)

Standardized canonical correlation coefficients for each of the variables are shown in Table B.2. The Wilks's lambda (indicating the degrees of overlap between the two distributions) was .5829. An eigenvalue of .686 was obtained, indicating that 69% of the variance was accounted for between the two groups, and the six variables accounted for 39.8% of the total variance.

Table B.2 Standardized Canonical Coefficients

Variable	Coefficient
History of falling	0.41111
Secondary diagnosis	0.41949
Ambulatory aid	0.49665
Intravenous therapy	0.50162
Gait	0.34784
Mental status	0.31223

3. Obtaining Scale Weights for Each Item

From the discriminant analysis output, the Fisher's linear function score was used to calculate the fall scale weights for each item. The score was obtained for each discriminant variable for both the fall and the control groups. As shown in Table B.3, values obtained for the control group were subtracted from the values obtained for the fall group for each item. For the scale to be optimally useful and for scores to be calculated easily, these values were then multiplied by 10 and brought to the nearest integer divisible by 5, provided that this procedure did not interfere with the discriminant values of the test. This technique ensured greater reliability than did the technique of improper linear modeling, where scale items are assigned equal values (Dawes, 1979) as is used, for example, in the Apgar scale (Apgar, 1953). These six items and values formed the Morse Fall Scale, with a maximum score of 125.[2]

Table B.3 Calculation of Scale Weights

	Fisher's Linear Functions Score			
Variable	Fall	Control	Fall-Control	Scale Value[3]
History of falling	2.6004	0.0704	2.6708	25
Secondary diagnosis	3.2857	1.7896	1.4961	15
Ambulatory aid	1.7458	0.3662	1.3795	15
Intravenous therapy	3.3969	1.1750	2.2219	20
Gait	1.3868	0.6230	0.7638	10
Mental status	1.0360	−0.3477	1.3837	15

4. Determining the Level of Risk

The constant obtained from the Fisher's linear score (again, the constant score for the fall group minus the score for the control group) is the score used to determine risk of falling, separating high risk from low risk. Next, using the SPSSx frequencies program (augmented with "select if" and "compute" statements), the constant score was adjusted by single increments. The analysis was then repeated with each increment, and the percentages of cases correctly and incorrectly identified with each solution were obtained. Increasing the constant (the level of determining risk) has the effect of decreasing the false positives while increasing false negatives, or vice versa if the constant is decreased. Because it was considered more important to reduce the number of false negatives (i.e., failing to identify a patient that was liable to fall) without greatly compromising the total percentage correct, the final selection of the constant was a matter of judgment (Dawes, 1979; Lachenbruch, 1975).[4]

5. Computer Testing of the Scale

Next, using SPSSx facilities, the data set was weighted to resemble the hospital population according to the patients' risk of falling in the institution. Because this institution had an average fall rate of 2.5 patient falls per 1,000 patient bed days, the probability of a fall was 1:40 during an average 30-day stay. Thus, the database was increased to include 100 cases from the fall group and 4,000 controls. The discriminant analysis procedures were then repeated in the normalized data set.

The result of the discriminant analysis with the "normalized" population (i.e., 100 fallers and 4,000 controls) classified 82.99% of the cases correctly, as follows:

	Actual Group	
Predicted Group	Fall	Control
Fall ($n = 100$)	78 (1.9%)	680 (16.59%)
Control ($n = 100$)	22 (0.54%)	3,320 (80.98%)

From the preceding data, the sensitivity of the scale, or the rate of a correct decision, is 78/100, or 78%. Thus, the positive predictive value is 78/(78 + 680) = 10.3%. Conversely, the specificity of the Scale, or the rate of correct decisions for patients who have not fallen, is 3,320/4,000 = 83%, and the negative predictive value is 3,320/ (22 + 3,320) = 99.2%.

6. Estimation of Reliability

Interrater reliability was established with 21 nurses rating six patients. To ensure consistency, patients' gaits were videotaped, and this videotape was used for the scoring. The interrater reliability estimation for a 5-item scale was $r = .96$ (see Note 4). Scores for individual items were history of falling and intravenous therapy, $r = 1.0$; secondary diagnosis, $r = .99$; ambulatory aids, $r = .98$; and gait, $r = .82$. A test for internal consistency revealed poor interitem correlations with a coefficient alpha of .16. This, combined with the results of analysis of variance, $F = 71.34, p < .0001$, suggests that the items are relatively independent. However, because the Scale is only six items long, this is perhaps a necessary feature for measuring a multifaceted phenomenon.

7. Establishment of Validity

When developing the scale, a major threat to validity was that the discriminatory power of the scale was tested on the same population from which the scale weights were obtained. This was remedied by randomly splitting the cases (using the nonnormalized data, $n = 200$) and repeating the scale construction procedures by obtaining scale weights from 50% of the cases and retesting the discriminatory power of these weights on the remaining 50% of the cases.

Validation of the scale by randomly splitting the data set did not alter the value of the weights obtained for the score variables. When tested on the remaining data ($n = 102$, 54 fallers and 48 controls), the percentage correctly classified by discriminant analysis was 79.41%. This change was not significant.

A second validation procedure was the examination of cases that were classified incorrectly by the discriminant analysis (i.e., the cases classified as false positive and false negative). These cases were traced in the original data, and the circumstances surrounding these falls were analyzed.

Examination of the 17 controls who were classified in the fall group (i.e., as false positives) showed that six of these patients (35%)

were disoriented, all 17 (100%) had difficulty with balance, and 16 of the 17 patients had an abnormal gait (three patients were rated as "weak" and 13 as "impaired"). Only three of these patients used walking aids, and one ambulated by leaning on the furniture. Ten weeks later, the charts of these patients were obtained from the record department and examined for the possibility of falls that may have occurred after data collection had been completed. In that period, three of the 17 patients had fallen (one patient three times) to give a total of five falls.

Twenty-two patients who had fallen were not classified in the fall group (i.e., were false negatives). Examination of these data showed that all patients were oriented, eight patients had a weak gait, and one had an impaired gait. Only one patient used a walking aid. Examination of the falls experienced by these patients permitted classification into two types of falls: the unanticipated physiological fall ($n = 8$) caused by "drop attacks," drug reactions, fainting, seizures, or patients with knees that "gave way," and the accidental fall ($n = 14$), which included patients who slipped, tripped, or "rolled out of bed" (see Morse et al., 1987).

A third method of validation was the prospective testing of the scale in three types of clinical settings: an acute care hospital (six units), long-term care (a psychogeriatric unit and a nursing home), and eight adult units in a rehabilitation hospital) (Morse, Black, Oberle, & Donahue, 1989). All patients ($n = 2,689$) were assessed daily for fall risk using the Morse Fall Scale. Differences in the distribution of scores were obtained by setting, with 19.6% scoring high risk of falling in the acute care area, 45.1% in the long-term care area, and 57.6% in the rehabilitation hospital. The Scale appeared sensitive to changes in the patients' conditions, with differences in the daily mean score between the long-stay and the short-stay patients and between surgical, medical, rehabilitation, and nursing home units.

In the study period, 147 falls were experienced by 107 patients. Of these falls, 6.8% of the patients scored as low risk of falling, 16.3% as moderate risk, and 76.9% as high risk of falling. Of these 147 falls, 61.9% were anticipated physiological falls (or falls that occur when the patient is disoriented, has a weak or impaired gait, and uses a walking aid), 20 (13.6%) were unanticipated falls (or falls that occur in patients who are usually oriented, who have drop attacks, or feel dizzy or faint), and 35 (24.5%) were scored as accidental falls (or falls that are caused when the patient slips, trips, or rolls out of bed). Of the 113 falls where the patients were rated as high risk of falling, 82 (72.6%) were anticipated physiological falls.

Notes

1. This research was conducted at a 1,200-bed urban hospital. Although primarily an acute care institution, the hospital also contained a 50-bed long-term geriatric center and a 140-bed Veterans' Home. Detailed statistics on falls occurring in the institution over the past 10 years showed a mean fall rate of 2.5 falls per 1,000 patient bed days. Thus, in this institution, a patient had a 1:400 chance of falling on any one day, or a 1:40 chance during an average 10-day period of hospitalization.

2. For ease of scoring, a simpler weighting system of assigning 1 if the attribute was present and 0 if the attribute was not present was tested. In this test, only 58% of the cases were classified correctly using discriminant analysis, or slightly better than would be obtained by chance alone.

3. Scale value was calculated as follows: Fall minus control multiplied by 10. The result was then rounded to the nearest integer divisible by 5.

4. This was calculated using the SPSSx statistical package and the following subroutine, where FC = falls correctly calculated; FR = falls correctly identified (true positive); FW = falls incorrectly identified (false negative); CW = control incorrectly identified (false positive); CR = controls correctly identified (true negative); TR = total percentage correct, VI group (1 = fall, 0 = control); VF = history of falling; VS = secondary diagnosis; VI = intravenous therapy; VM = mental status; VA = ambulatory aides used; and VG = gait.

```
COMPUTE FC=25*VF+15*VS+15*VA+20*VI+10*VG+15*VM-(constant score)
COMPUTE FR=0
COMPUTE FW=0
COMPUTE CW=0
COMPUTE CR=0
COMPUTE TR=0
IF (VI EQ 0 AND FC GT 0) FR=1
IF (VI EQ 0 AND FC LE 0) FW=1
IF (VI EQ 1 AND FC LE 0) CR=1
IF (FR EQ 1 OR CR EQ 1) TR=1
FREQUENCIES GENERAL=V1 FR FW CW CR TR/
```

5. Reprinted with permission from *Canadian Journal on Aging, 8*, 366-377.

Endnote

Given that the scores on the Morse Fall Scale increase with age
(see Figure B.1), and age is often considered a significant variable on
other scales, why did age not load as a significant variable? It is thought
that the risk factors associated with age were accounted for in other
variables, such as gait, history of falling, walking aids, and mental
status.

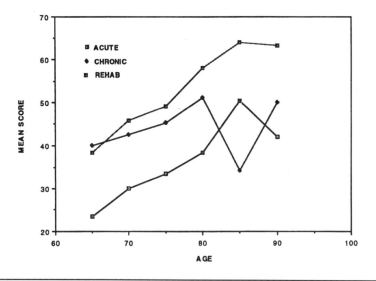

Figure B.1. Mean Score for Age in Three Different Settings

Appendix C

The Morse Fall Scale:
Determining Level of Risk

When using the *Morse Fall Scale*, the *level of risk* that determines the percentage of patients who will receive preventive strategies must be adjusted to suit the patient population. Because health care institutions usually are sorted into units and according to level of care and patient diagnoses, the risk of falling varies markedly from area to area. For instance, in an acute surgical ward, where the average length of stay is usually less than 120 days and the patients are ambulatory shortly following surgery, the number of falls reported in that unit is less than a geriatric medical unit, and the mean fall score for the unit would be lower than the mean score for the geriatric unit.

This variation poses a problem when determining the high-risk score for the institution. If the score is set low enough to detect all the possible falls in the surgical unit (e.g., 25), then almost all of the patients in the medical unit will score above 25. This will result in the nurses having to declare all the geriatric medical patients at high risk of falling—in short, the scale loses its "discriminating power" and, because some patients are more likely to fall than others, will give too many false positives (see Morse, 1986).

Selecting a uniform higher value does not solve the problem, because then on the surgical wards, patients who are likely to fall will be judged not at risk (i.e., the scale will give too many false negatives). Thus, determining the score that will indicate high risk must be determined *by unit* in institutions where the patient population is diverse.

Administrators must recognize that setting the scale too low, too conservatively is costly because fall prevention strategies will be implemented as a result of too many false negatives—that is, for patients who are less likely to fall. Nurses will consider the scale obscure and will not bother to use it at all. Setting the level of risk at too high a level will result in patients being unprotected, falling, and injuring themselves—that is, there will be too many false negatives.

A second consideration is that the mathematical solution may not be the optimal clinical solution, because the mathematical model does not consider the ethical-moral consequences of an incorrect decision of the risk of injury to unprotected patients.

Calculating Risk

Method 1

The first principle is to recognize that the scale does not predict all fallers with 100% accuracy. The scale will predict only 82.9% of fallers, the anticipated physiological falls from a normal hospital population. When these data are placed on a graph and the level of high risk moved above 25, the percentage of false negatives (i.e., fallers who will be classified as nonfallers) increases (see Figure C.1). However, the percentage of nonfallers identified as at risk of falling will decrease. Conversely, if the level of risk score is moved toward zero, all the falls will be detected (i.e., the false negatives will not be a problem), but a high percentage of nonfallers will be classified as fall prone (i.e., the percentage of false positives will increase).

Method 2

The method is a more subjective one, often preferred by clinicians. The steps are as follows:

1. Score all patients in the unit.
2. List the scores by increment. For example, in a 34-bed surgical unit, the services may appear as shown in Table C.1.

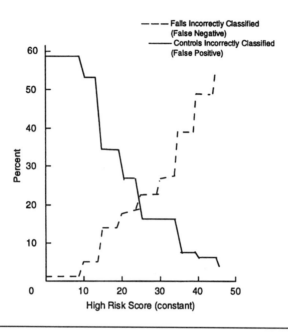

Figure C.1. Number of Falls and Controls Incorrectly Classified for Different Settings of the Scale

The staff may elect to set the high score at 25, in which case 38% of the patients would be scoring not at risk, and fall prevention strategies would be implemented for 62% of the patients scoring at risk. However, the range of scores is large, and they may wish to "set" risk at two levels: medium and high. In this case, medium risk may be 25 to 45 (13 patients) and high risk, above 45 (8 patients).

Variation in the distribution of scores by acute care, long-term care, or rehabilitation setting are presented in Appendix E, Table E.2, and may be used as a reference for determining the cutoff score. Note that in the total scores for this study, 52.5% of the scores were 25 or below, yet in the long-term care setting, only 20.1% of the scores were in this range.

Table C.1 Distribution of Fall Scores in a Sample Unit

Fall Scores	Number of Patients	Cumulative %
0	6	18
10	2	24
15	3	32
20	2	38
25	2	44
30	3	53
35	5	68
40	1	71
45	2	76
50	2	82
55	1	85
60	1	88
65	0	88
70	1	91
75	1	94
80	0	94
85	1	97
90	0	97
95	1	100
100	0	
105	0	
110	0	
115	0	
120	0	

Valuing the Cost of an Incorrect Decision

As stated, administrators also must consider the cost of a fall prevention program on hospital resources. Setting the at-risk score too high will result in fallers being classified as nonfallers, and if an injury occurs, it will legally jeopardize the institution. If, on the other hand, setting the risk score too low will result in too many patients at very low risk of falling being classified at high risk of falling, it will result in wasted staff time, and it will place the fall prevention program in jeopardy. Staff will rightly consider use of the fall scale "silly" if all patients are going to be rated at risk.

Table C.2 Hypothesized Costs to the Institution[a] Based on Various
Estimations of Risk

	Hypothesized Weight				
Cost Plan	Fall Group Correctly Identified	Fall Group Identified as Controls	Controls Correctly Identified	Controls Identified as Fallers	Level of Scale for High Risk at Minimum Cost
COST 1	0	+10	0	+1	35
COST 2	0	+50	0	+1	25
COST 3	0	+100	0	+1	0

a. Estimated using a normalized population of 100 falls and 4,000 controls.

Yet there is another consideration. The consequences of not
identifying a faller as fall prone, therefore risking injury and legal
liability, may be considered 10 times (or 20 times—the number is
determined by the institution) worse than identifying a nonfaller as a
faller. The former has human costs and possible legal costs, whereas
the latter may have high staff time. This is the relative risk, and it is
used to weight the group at risk.

These cost plans are shown in Table C.2. COST 1: the hypothesized group—a fall correctly identified and a control correctly identified—was weighted as 0, not identifying a fall was weighted as +10,
and a control identified as a faller as +1. This resulted in an increase
in the minimal level of setting the risk score.

These cost models may be plotted further for various scores, as
shown in Figure C.2. Note that there is a best minimum cost for each
model. For COST 1, this is 25-39, so a high risk score of 35 should
be used. For the second cost estimation, where the cost of not
identifying a fall-prone patient (false negative) is estimated at 50 times
that of identifying a nonfaller as a faller, the minimum high-risk score
is 25. But if the estimated cost is 200 times greater for a false negative,
the minimum cost is zero, and all patients must be considered at risk
of falling.

In summary, to retain the discriminatory power of the scale, the
risk score should be adjusted according to the patient population and

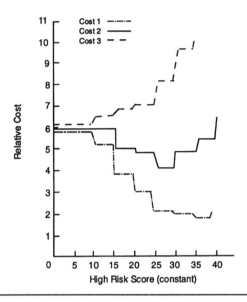

Figure C.2. Cost Estimates for Three Models With Different Settings of the High Risk Score (i.e., Constant)

the cost that administrators place on not identifying a fall. Previous scales have not been developed to identify the fall-prone patient in high-risk areas, such as long-term care. In geriatric or rehabilitation areas, all patients have scored "at risk of falling"; thus, the usefulness of identifying patients at risk is lost. In reality, all of these patients are at risk of falling. However, as clinicians are aware, some patients are more at risk than others, and therefore, although precautions may be made with all patients, relative risk also may be measured and extra precautions targeted toward those patients most at risk.

Note: Reprinted with permission from *Canadian Journal of Public Health*, 77 (Suppl. 1), 21-25.

Appendix D

A Comparison of Methods of Calculating Fall Rates

Fall rates have been difficult to compare because there has not been an established standard for reporting fall statistics. Without such a standard, hospitals have been forced to use a variety of different reporting conventions. In this appendix, the various methods of reporting fall statistics and the strengths and limitations of each method are discussed. Data used in this analysis were obtained from a prospective study that examined the identification of fall-prone patients in three settings—acute care, long-term care, and rehabilitation—in two institutions (Morse & Morse, 1988). The rates for the acute care institution were obtained from six patient care units (medical and surgical) where the patients were considered at a higher risk of falling than was the total hospital population. Therefore, these rates are higher than normally reported. The long-term care sample consisted of one psychogeriatric unit and one 75-bed unit in a male nursing home. The rehabilitation sample was obtained from eight adult units in a rehabilitation hospital. Data for these three settings were collected for 6 months, from November 1985 to April 1986. Historical controls, obtained from hospital records for the same period in the previous year, are presented for comparative purposes. Table D.1 presents the data from this study.

Table D.1 Data Obtained From a Prospective Study Examining the Identification of Fall-Prone Patients in Three Settings

Variables for Study Period (1986) and Previous Year (1985)[a]	*Data Used in Analysis of Fall Rates*			
	Area			
	Acute Care (n)	Long-Term Care (n)	Rehabilitation (n)	Total (N)
Patient falls				
1985	55	35	52	142
1986	48	41	58	147
Patients who fell[b]				
1986	39	25	39	103
Patients who were injured				
1986	13	8	20	41
Patients at risk				
1986	1,939	24	626	2,689
Patient bed days				
1985	16,380	13,413	17,796	47,589
1986	16,563	13,542	19,841	49,946
Mean length of stay (days)				
1986	10	—	40	N/A

a. For a 6-month period, and includes repeated falls by the same patient.
b. One fall recorded per patient.

1. Patient Fall Rates

Health care institutions calculate the patient fall rate as

$$\frac{\text{number of patient falls}}{\text{number of patient bed days}} \times 1{,}000$$

Data are collected over a set period of time. Note that *all falls* are included in this formula, not all *patients who have fallen,* so that repeated falls experienced by the same patient are included in the numerator. Using data from Table D.1, the fall rates for these three settings can be calculated as 2.9 per 1,000 patient bed days for the acute care institutions, 2.92 for the rehabilitation hospital, and 3.0 for the long-term care area. The fall rate for the three areas combined is 2.94 per 1,000 patient bed days.

2. The Number of Patients at Risk

The second most commonly used statistic is the

$$\frac{\text{number of patient falls}}{\text{number of patients at risk}} \times 1{,}000$$

Because all institutionalized patients theoretically are at risk of falling, the number of patients at risk equals the number of patients admitted during the study regardless of their length of stay. "At risk" in this context does not refer to risk factors contributing to a fall. This method, as with the patient fall rate, includes the multiple, or repeated, falls of any patient in the numerator. This may inflate the statistics artificially if there is a patient on the unit who falls frequently. The inclusion of multiple falls may give unstable or fluctuating rates over time. This is particularly important if falls are being monitored over a short period of time, such as when the administrator is working with monthly totals. Using the statistic from Table D.1 for 1986, we have the following:

$$\frac{147}{2{,}689} \times 1{,}000 = 54.67 \text{ per } 1{,}000$$

Note that if a unit sometimes has a patient who falls repeatedly, and if the unit uses this statistic over a short period of time, such as the monthly monitoring of the unit, then this statistic may provide very unstable results. Differences between the *number of patient falls* and the *number of patients who fall* should be evident.

3. The Number of Patients Who Fell

When the *number of patients who fell* is used as the numerator, rather than the *number of falls* per se, the fall rate is:

$$\frac{103}{2{,}689} = 38.3 \text{ per } 1{,}000$$

4. The Number of Falls per Bed

This statistic is as follows:

$$\frac{\text{number of patient falls per time period}}{\text{number of beds}}$$

The potential problem with this method is that it gives no information about the length of time that the patients are at risk and is based on the unrealistic assumption of a 100% occupancy rate. Therefore, this statistic is dependent on the characteristics of the patient population, and it is of limited use for comparison between units. For example, if the institution has long-stay patients, one would get results similar to the *number of patients at risk* if there was no patient turnover during the study period. On the other hand, if used for an acute care unit with short-stay patients, there would be a large discrepancy between these two results. Also note that *all falls* are included in this formula, not just the *number of patients who have fallen.*

5. The Probability of Falling

This formula is useful because it estimates the probability of any one patient falling on any one day:

$$\frac{\text{Fall rate}}{1,000}$$

Thus, based on the rehabilitation rate of 2.9 per 1,000 patient bed days, there is a 1:345 chance of a patient falling on any given day.

The reason that the formula yields only an estimate of probability has to do with more than just sampling variability. Because the falls counted in the fall rate include those from multiple fallers, patients who have been counted only once will be calculated to have a higher fall probability than should be the case.

If one wishes to calculate the probability of falling during an average hospital stay, it is not quite accurate to multiply the probability for a single day by the number of days' stay. (If the duration were long enough, such a calculation would produce a "probability" greater than 1, which is meaningless.) The correct calculation is done by subtracting the probability from 1 to get the chances of not falling per day, then raising that value to the power given by the number of days, and finally subtracting the result from 1 again.

Thus, in the rehabilitation unit, with a fall probability of 0.0029 and a mean stay of 40 days, we would calculate:

$$[1 - (1 - .0029)^{40}] = [1 - .9971^{40}] = [1 - .8903] = 0.11,$$

which means that there is about an 11% chance of falling during a stay in the rehabilitation unit.

Note: Reprinted with permission from *Quality Review Bulletin: Journal of Quality Assurance*, *14*(12), 369-371.

Appendix E

Prospective Testing of the Morse Fall Scale[1]

The purpose of this study was to clinically validate the *Morse Fall Scale* in three types of patient care areas (acute medical and surgical units, long term care areas, and a rehabilitation hospital). Patients' fall risk was rated daily and falls that occurred were analyzed by type of fall and risk score to determine the feasibility of using the *Scale* in practice.

Method

Setting

The study was conducted in two institutions. Six units were selected from the acute care division (general surgical [2 units], ophthalmology [1 unit] and 3 medical units) along with 2 units from the long term care division (psychogeriatric and nursing home) from a 1,100 bed general hospital. Also eight adult units were selected from the 240 bed rehabilitation hospital (i.e., neuromuscular, orthopedic, diabetes, weight control, head injury [2 units] and a CVA unit). The average length of stay in the acute care areas of the acute care hospital was 10 days, with a fall rate of 2.5 falls per 1,000 patient bed days in the previous year. Patients were frequently transferred to the rehabilitation hospital from other hospitals in the region, and the average length of stay in that hospital was 40 days. The patient fall rate for the rehabilitation hospital for the previous year was 3.2 falls per 1,000 patient bed days.

Research Design

A pilot project to assess the feasibility of the project was initiated in November, 1985. The pilot was conducted for two weeks to determine the most effective methods of data collection. Thereafter, one unit in each institution was introduced to the project every few weeks. For the first one or two weeks, staff were introduced to the project, instructed in the use of the *Morse Fall Scale* (from a video learning tape) and fall-prevention strategies were discussed. Nurses rated all patients' risk of falling daily, documented fall prevention strategies used and, if a fall occurred, noted the time of occurrence, type of fall and any causative factors. Only falls that occurred on the patient's unit were included in the analysis (i.e., patient falls that occurred in another department, such as x-ray, or while the patient was out on a pass, were excluded).

Results

Data collection extended from December 1, 1985 to April 30, 1986. A total of 252 weeks of data were collected from 16 patient care units. 2,689 patients were assessed during this period, 41.2% of whom were over the age of 65 years; pediatric patients were excluded.[2] Patients are shown in Table E.1, by unit and sex. A total of 49,946 patient bed days were recorded: 16,563 from the acute care areas, 13,542 from the long term care areas, and 19,841 from the rehabilitation hospital. As patients usually were not discharged from hospital until they could cope without surveillance, the mean length of stay in each institution was used as an indication to compare the short and the long stay patients. The mean length of stay was 10 days in the acute care hospital and 40 days in the rehabilitation hospital. However, the mean length of stay could not be calculated for the long term care area as the patients are rarely discharged.

Table E.1 Patient Gender by Unit

Unit	Male n	Male %	Female n	Female %	Total n	Total %
Acute care						
Ophthalmology	143	49.1	148	50.9	291	10.8
General surgery I	115	49.8	116	50.2	231	8.6
General surgery II	146	54.7	121	45.3	267	9.9
General medicine I	260	54.5	217	45.5	477	17.7
General medicine II	139	59.4	95	40.6	234	8.7
G.I. and endocrinology	205	46.7	234	53.3	439	16.3
Long-Term						
Long-term care	13	28.3	33	71.7	46	1.7
Nursing home	78	100.0	0	0.0	78	2.9
Rehabilitation						
Neuromuscular	19	44.2	24	55.8	43	1.6
Head injury I	15	16.7	75	83.3	90	3.3
Orthopedics	84	94.4	5	5.6	89	3.3
Diabetes	39	60.0	26	40.0	65	2.4
Weight control	28	31.5	61	68.5	89	3.3
Head injury II	25	39.7	38	60.3	63	2.3
Stroke I	50	37.3	84	62.7	134	5.0
Stroke II	35	66.0	18	34.0	53	2.0
Total	1,394	51.8	1,295	48.2	2,689	100.0

Of 2,689 patients in both institutions, 1,265 (47.1%) scored as low risk of falling (i.e., ≤ 20), 734 (27.3%) scored as medium risk (i.e., 25-40) and 690 (25.5%) as high risk (i.e., ≥ 45). The distribution of total fall scores obtained by setting are shown in Table E.2. Distinct differences in the distribution of scores between groups were immediately apparent. The mean score in the acute care setting was 24.78 (*s.d.* 22.95), with 58.3% scoring as low risk, 21.8% as medium risk and 19.6% as a high risk. In the long term care setting, a mean score of 44.37 was obtained (*s.d.* 23.35), and 20.1% of these patients received a low score, 34.7% a medium score and 45.1% a high score. The scores for the rehabilitation area, with a mean of 41.9% (*s.d.* 21.11), showed that 15.6% rated low, 25.8% medium and 57.6% as a high risk.

Table E.2 Fall Scores by Setting

Fall Score	Acute Care		Long-Term Care		Rehabilitation		Total		
	n	%	n	%	n	%	n	%	Cumulative %
0	522	26.9	3	2.4	27	4.3	552	20.5	20.5
10	37	1.9	0	0.0	14	2.2	51	1.9	22.4
15	241	12.4	22	17.7	57	9.1	320	11.9	34.3
20	332	17.1	0	0.0	10	1.6	342	12.7	47.0
25	63	3.2	4	3.2	81	12.9	148	5.5	52.5
30	99	5.1	11	8.9	22	3.5	132	4.9	57.4
35	197	10.2	16	12.9	49	7.8	262	9.7	67.1
40	66	3.4	12	9.7	114	18.2	192	7.1	74.2
45	75	3.9	0	0.0	6	1.0	81	3.0	77.2
50	75	3.9	17	13.7	91	14.5	183	6.8	84.0
55	41	2.1	1	0.8	15	2.4	57	2.1	86.1
60	45	2.3	7	5.6	26	4.2	78	2.9	89.0
65	20	1.0	9	7.3	39	6.2	68	2.5	91.5
70	35	1.8	0	0.0	2	0.3	37	1.4	92.9
75	25	1.3	13	10.5	52	8.3	90	3.4	96.3
80	7	0.4	1	0.8	6	1.0	14	0.5	96.5
85	20	1.0	0	0.0	0	0.0	20	0.7	97.5
90	6	0.3	7	5.6	13	2.1	26	1.0	98.5
95	13	0.7	0	0.0	1	0.2	14	0.5	99.0
100	6	0.3	0	0.0	0	0.0	6	0.2	99.2
105	3	0.2	1	0.8	1	0.2	5	0.2	99.4
110	5	0.3	0	0.0	0	0.0	5	0.2	99.6
115	0	0.0	0	0.0	0	0.0	0	0.0	99.6
120	0	0.0	0	0.0	0	0.0	0	0.0	99.6
125	1	0.1	0	0.0	0	0.0	1	0.0	99.6
Missing	5	0.3	0	0.0	0	0.0	5	0.2	99.8
Total	1,939	100.1	124	99.9	626	100.0	2,689	99.8	100.0

Analysis of each item in the Morse Fall Scale showed that 50.4% of the patients' scores varied during the hospital stay. The items that increase the mean scores were attributed to changes in ambulatory aids (30.1%) and deterioration in gait from normal to weak, or weak to impaired (23.4%). A fall increased the patient scores in only 12% of the cases. On the other hand, a decrease in patient scores resulted from improvement in gait in 43.1% of the cases, the removal of an IV in 23.9%, and an improvement in mental status in 18.1%. In the acute care setting, differences in fall scores according to patient condition were reflected when the scores of the short stay (i.e., ≤ 10 days) and the long stay (> 10 days) patients were compared. When analyzed day by day, changes in the patients' scores reflected differences in the patients' condition (see Figure E.1). For example, many patients are admitted to the eye unit for minor surgery. The pattern of patient scores in this unit peak on the day following surgery (Day 2) for those admitted for minor surgery, and the scores decrease when these patients begin to ambulate as they approach discharge. On the other hand, the scores remain elevated for longer term patients. Unfortunately, the mean length of stay of 40 days did not provide an adequate sample to permit analysis between long and short stay patients in the rehabilitation hospital or for the long-term care setting. However, daily patient scores in the rehabilitation hospital did increase the second day after admission, perhaps because the patients after assessment were no longer on bed rest and were encouraged to ambulate. Nevertheless, in both the rehabilitation and the long-term care areas, scores were relatively flat compared with the variability evident in the acute care hospital.

Examination of the type of patient fall (i.e., physiological anticipated fall, physiological unanticipated fall, and accidental fall) by the patients' fall scores revealed that of 147 falls, 91 (i.e., 61.9%) were physiological anticipated falls; whereas only 20 (13.6%) were unanticipated falls and 36 (24.5%) were accidental. The largest percentage of fallers, regardless of type, were high scorers (76.9%); this difference was particularly apparent in the anticipated physiological fall category. The association between fall score category and type of fall was statistically significant ($\chi^2 = 30.2$, d.f. = 4, p < .01) (see Table E.3). On the other hand, most of the falls with patient scores in the low or moderate categories were classified as "unanticipated" or "accidental" falls.

Of the patients who fell and were injured, the greatest proportion of injuries were incurred by those patients scored as "anticipated

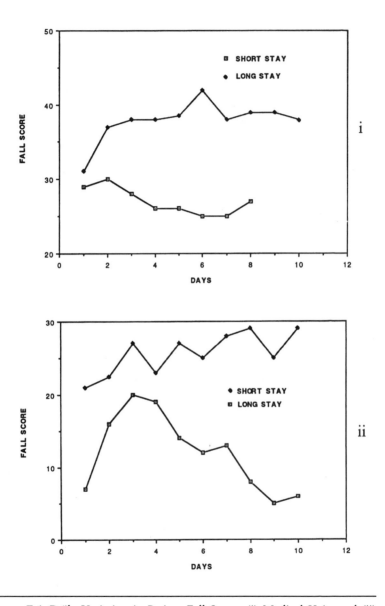

Figure E.1 Daily Variation in Patient Fall Scores (i) Medical Units and (ii) Surgical Units

Table E.3 Falls Score by Type of Fall and Setting

Fall Score	Anticipated (n = 91)[a]			Unanticipated (n = 20)[a]			Accidental (n = 36)[a]			Total	
	A/C[b]	LTC[c]	R[d]	A/C	LTC	R	A/C	LTC	R	n	%
Low	0	0	1	5	0	0	2	1	1	10	6.8
Moderate	4	2	2	1	1	3	2	5	4	24	16.3
High	26	25	31	3	1	6	5	6	10	113	76.9
Total	30	27	34	9	2	9	9	12	15	147[e]	100.0

a. Number of falls.
b. Acute care.
c. Long-term care.
d. Rehabilitation.
e. Includes repeated falls (n = 107 patients).

Table E.4 Injuries by Score and Type of Fall

Fall Score	Anticipated (n = 91)[a]	Unanticipated (n = 20)[a]	Accidental (n = 36)[a]	Total (n = 147)[a]
Low	0	2 minor	2 minor	4
Moderate	1 serious[b]	3 minor	3 minor	7
High	13 minor 8 serious[d]	5 minor	1 serious[c] 3 minor	30
Total	22	10	9	41

a. Number of falls.
b. One fractured ankle.
c. Two fractured ribs; one fractured hip; one fractured ankle; one fractured vertebrae (C2);
   one laceration; one sprain; one concussion.
d. One fractured hip and elbow.

physiological falls" (i.e., 22 of 91 falls, or 24.2%). 8 of these 22 falls resulted in serious injuries (see Table E.4). The only other serious injury in the study was an accidental fall, also experienced by a patient with a high fall score, who fractured both a hip and an elbow. 13 patients from the acute care area, 8 from the long term care and 20 from the rehabilitation areas received injuries resulting from falls.

Table E.5 Numbers of Patients Who Fell Repeatedly, by Setting and Number of Falls

Number of Falls	Setting			
	Acute Care	Long-Term Care	Rehabilitation	
2	7	5	6	
3	1	0	2	
4	0	2	2	
5	0	1	0	*
Total	17	23	26	= 66

Repeat Fallers

During the study period, 26 patients fell twice or more for a total of 66 falls (i.e., 26 first falls and 40 repeated falls), with one patient falling 5 times in the study period. The numbers of falls by patient care area are shown in Table E.5. The mean fall score for patients in this category was 80 (*s.d.* 17.6).

All of the scores of patients who fell repeatedly in the rehabilitation hospital are shown by fall in Table E.6. In this group, the scores of 6 of the 10 patients increased considerably over the course of hospitalization. 3 of the patients in the acute care hospital also had increased scores with subsequent falls, but the patients in the long term areas, with higher mean scores, tended to have scores that were more stable.

At the conclusion of the project, the nursing staff were surveyed to ascertain the clinical feasibility of continuing the use of the Scale. 175 nurses responded, of whom 82.9% rated the Scale as quick and easy to use, and 54% estimated that it took less than three minutes to rate a patient using the Scale. 63% thought it should be a part of ongoing nursing assessment.

Table E.6 Fall Scores for Patients Who Fell Repeatedly:
Rehabilitation Hospital

Patient	First	Second	Third	Fourth
		Fall		
1	50^a	105^a		
2	90^a	90^a		
3	65^{ab}	90^{ab}		
4	35^b	75^b		
5	75^b	75^b		
6	25^b	40^b		
7	75	75^{ab}	75^{ab}	
8	75^b	75	75^b	
9	60^b	60^b	90^b	90
10	40^b	65^b	75^b	90

a. Same circumstances at time of fall (e.g., going to the bathroom).
b. Same activity at time of fall (e.g., transferring or reaching for an object).

Discussion

Longitudinal evaluation of the *Morse Fall Scale* shows that the Scale appears to be a valid predictor of patient falls. Of the total of 107 patients who fell during the study period, 113 of the falls were experienced by the 75 patients who scored in the "high risk" category. The Scale was particularly successful in predicting anticipated physiological falls; 90.1% of fallers in this category were identified by the *Scale* as being at high risk. Furthermore, the Scale is sensitive to changes in the patient condition, as evidenced by the variability in daily scores, particularly in the surgical areas of the acute care hospital. Items that contribute to the patients' fall scores vary by unit (i.e., by medical specialty), which suggests that the Scale is sensitive to levels of disability. There are distinct differences in the score profiles according to institution, with a greater proportion of patients receiving a high score in the long-term care institution and the rehabilitation hospital. Thus, the Scale is correctly identifying differences that are intuitively obvious; one would expect rehabilitation and long-term care patients to be at greater risk of falling.

It is important to note that although more than 57.6% of the rehabilitation hospital patients scored as having a high risk of falling, the fall rate (2.7 falls per 1,000 patient bed days) was lower than the long-term care area and the acute care area (3.0 and 2.9 falls per 1,000 patient bed days respectively). All but one of the serious injuries occurring during the study period were in patients who were identified by the Fall Scale as being at high risk of falling. This suggests that patients in the high risk category are more likely to be injured if they do fall and indicates that those caring for the patients with a high fall score should be increasingly aware of the necessity of fall prevention.

Examination of the scores of the patients that fell repeatedly showed that the scores were very high, and in 9 cases, the scores increased substantially with each successive fall, indicating increasing frailty. This is consistent with other research (Gryfe, Aimes, & Ashley, 1977) which notes that falls tend to cluster prior to death.

There were two limitations in this study. Firstly, the patient care areas were not selected randomly. They were chosen because they were considered "high risk" areas where patient falls were problematic. Thus, areas such as obstetrics were excluded, and the sample was not representative of a typical hospital population. Patients under the age of 18 years were also excluded, and no data are available on children or younger adolescents. It is recommended that the study be repeated, and all patients in several institutions be scored so that more representative norms of patient scores may be obtained.

The second limitation is a problem that is unavoidable when studying patient falls, and it is related to research design. It is not feasible to separate the rating of fall risk from the subsequent possibility of a fall without also trying simultaneously to prevent the fall. Thus, the researcher is in a paradoxical situation of both predicting the criterion variable and preventing its occurrence. There is, however, no moral solution to this problem, and it becomes a choice of conducting imperfect research or not conducting the research at all (Robb, Stegman, & Wolanin, 1986). Thus, the staff were given fall prevention strategies to prevent falls in patients rated at medium or high risk of falling despite the fact that successfully preventing a fall could interfere with the significance of the results.

A related problem with the researcher's or administrator's sudden interest in falls is the increased reporting of falls during a study period. As all patient falls that result in injury are reported, it is probable that injury rate is less variable to reporting error than fall rate. It is recommended that in future studies the injury rate during the research period be compared with previous years to identify changes in the standards of reporting.

Nevertheless, the major strengths of this project were that the study was conducted in the clinical areas, during normal working days, and the ratings were done by clinicians who would normally be using the *Scale*. As other fall scales have been too complex to use without pencil and paper (Rainville, 1984), required a physical examination (Tideiksaar & Kay, 1986) or taking a clinical history (Patel, 1976) to assess the patient's fall risk, the ease of use and administrative feasibility of the Morse Fall Scale appears advantageous. However, although the Scale assists in the prediction of fall-prone patients, investigation of methods to prevent patient falls must continue.

Notes

1. Reprinted with permission from Pergamon Press. Taken from Morse, J. M., Black, C., Oberle, K., & Donahue, P. (1989). A prospective study to identify the fall-prone patient. *Social Science & Medicine, 28*(1), 81-86.
2. Those patients under 18 years of age were excluded from the research project because (1) regulation for the protection of Human Subjects requires parental consent for the inclusion of minors in research and (2) falls by young children include falls from climbing and tripping which are a part of normal activity and thus are considered a separate phenomenon.

Appendix F

Resources

Using the Morse Fall Scale Training Video

A 10-minute videotape on the use of the Morse Fall Scale is available from:

Educational Audiovisual Services
Glenrose Rehabilitation Hospital
10230-111 Avenue
Edmonton, Alberta T5G 0B7
CANADA   Phone: (403) 471-2262

Restraint-Free Environment

<u>Resources and Consultation</u>

Untie the Elderly
Kendall Corporation
P.O. Box 100
Kennet Square, PA 19348   Phone: (215) 388-7001

Patient Alarms[1]

Pressure-sensitive alarms usually include a monitor or control unit and some type of pressure-sensitive pad or strip that is positioned under the patient. As the pressure is released or varied, the alarm sounds. Units can sound at bedside and/or the nurses' station through the nurse call system. Various adjustments can be made by nurses to tailor these systems to the patient's needs, including alarm time delay, mute settings, or weight sensitivity. Portable units use disposable sensor pads; however, permanently installed units are also available.

For more information on pressure-sensitive alarms, contact:

Bed-Check Corporation
P.O. Box 170
Tulsa, OK 74101

Alarm: Bed-Check and
　　　　Chair-Check
Phone: (800) 523-7956

Hill-Rom
1069 State Route 46E
Batesville, IN 47006

Alarm: Bed Exit System

Phone: (800) 445-3730

Posey Company
5635 Peck Road
Arcadia, CA 91006-0020

Alarm: Posey Sitter

Phone: (800) 447-6739

RF Technologies, Inc.
3125 N. 126th Street
Brookfield, WI 53005

Alarm: Code Alert Bed/
　　　　Chair Alarm
Phone: (800) 669-9946

Stryker Medical
6300 Sprinkle Road
Kalamazoo, MI 49001-9799

Alarm: Bed Exit Alarm

Phone: (800) 669-4968

Tactilitics, Inc.   Alarm: RN+ Systems
5595 Arapahoe Road
Boulder, CO 80303   Phone: (800) 866-4544

Tapeswitch Corporation   Alarm: Nurse Alert
100 Schmitt Boulevard
Farmingdale, NY 11735   Phone: (516) 694-6312

Magnetized sensor alarms sound when a magnet is disconnected from the control unit as the patient moves beyond the range of the connecting line. The connecting line is secured to the patient's clothing, to the bed linens, or even across a door. When the line is extended beyond its length, the magnet is disconnected from the control unit and the alarm rings. Units are portable, and the length of the connecting line can be adjusted to meet the patient's individual needs for monitoring.

For more information on magnetized sensor alarms, contact:

Alert Care, Inc.   Alarm: Tether Alarm
591 Redwood Hwy.
Suite 2125
Mill Valley, CA 94940   Phone: (800) 826-7444

Posey Company   Alarm: Posey Personal Alarm
5635 Peck Road
Arcadia, CA 91006-0020   Phone: (800) 447-6739

Wander Guard, Inc.   Alarm: TABS Mobility Monitors
PO Box 80238
Lincoln, NE 68501-0238   Phone: (800) 824-2996

Patient-worn movement detectors are positioned on the patient's leg (worn above the knee) so that movement to a near-vertical position is detected. The alarm sounds from the control unit on the patient device. The control units are attached to the patient-worn device, which is patient specific and can be laundered.

For more information on patient-worn movement detectors, contact:

Alert Care, Inc.   Alarm: Ambularm
591 Redwood Hwy.
Suite 2125
Mill Valley, CA 94940   Phone: (800) 826-7444

Restraining devices are available in various forms. Some systems employ physical restraints along with an alarm device that sounds when the restraint is pulled to maximum distance.

For more information on restraining devices, contact:

FSM Corporation   Alarm: Fallsafe Monitor
20 Oakshore Drive
Bratenahl, OH 44108   Phone: (800) 923-7233

Posey Company
5635 Peck Road
Arcadia, CA 91006-0020   Phone: (800) 447-6739

Note

1. This section was compiled to provide both an overview of the types of alarms currently available and contact information for further inquiries regarding the products. This listing is not meant to imply an endorsement of the products' safety or effectiveness and is not exhaustive.

Additional References

General/Comprehensive

Downton, J. H. (1993). *Falls in the elderly.* London: Edward Arnold.
Tideiksaar, R. (1993). *Falls in older persons: Prevention and management in hospitals and nursing homes.* Boulder, CO: Tactilitics.

Fall Assessment

Andriola, M. (1978). When an elderly patient complains of weakness. *Geriatrics, 33,* 79-85.
Ashley, M., Gryfe, C., & Amies, A. (1977). A longitudinal study of falls in an elderly population: Circumstances of falling. *Age and Ageing, 4,* 211-220.
Ashton, J., Gilbert, D., Hayward, G., O'dell, C., & Rogowski, B. (1989). Predicting patient falls in an acute care nursing setting. *Kansas Nurse, 64*(10), 3-5.
Baker, L. (1992). Developing a safety plan that works for patients and nurses. *Rehabilitation Nursing, 17,* 264-266.
Barbieri, E. G. (1983). Patient falls are not patient accidents. *Journal of Gerontological Nursing, 3,* 165-173.
Barrowclough, F. (1979). Danger! Why old people fall. *Nursing Mirror, 148,* 28-29.
Bartlett, S., Maki, B., Fernie, G., & Halliday, P. (1986). On the classification of a geriatric subject as a faller or non-faller. *Medical and Biological Engineering and Computing, 24,* 219-222.
Botez, M. I. (1982). Falls. *British Journal of Hospital Medicine, 28,* 494-503.
Bright, M., Minny, L., Ratsey, G., & Rawstorne, S. (1983). Patients who fall in hospital: Contributing factors. *South African Journal of Nursing, 1,* 52-54.
Brocklehurst, J., Robertson, D., & James-Groom, P. (1982). Clinical correlates of sway in old age—sensory modalities. *Age and Ageing, 11,* 1-10.
Brownlee, M. G., Banks, M. A., Crosbie, W. J., Meldrum, F., & Nimmo, M. A. (1989). Consideration of spatial orientation mechanisms as related to elderly fallers. *Gerontology, 35,* 323-331.
Campbell, M. (1988). Risk management and an evaluation of patient falls. *Dimensions in Health Service, 65*(5), 26-27.
Castellsagué, R. M., Elorza, C., Perez-Company, P., & Abello, C. (1989). Nursing quality assurance in Spain: Two experiences. *Australian Clinical Review, 9*(2), 86-90.

Chipman, C. (1981). What does it mean when a patient falls? Part I: Pinpointing the cause. *Geriatrics, 36*(9), 83-85.

Cohen, T. E., & Lasley, D. (1985). Visual depth illusion and falls in the elderly. *Clinics in Geriatric Medicine, 1,* 601-620.

Costa, A. J. (1991). Preventing falls in your elderly patients. *Postgraduate Medicine, 89*(1), 139-142.

Coyle, N. (1979). A problem-focused approach to nursing audit: Patient falls. *Cancer Nursing, 79,* 389-391.

Craft, G. (1979). Patient safety programs: A possible solution. *Bulletin of the American College of Surgeons, 5,* 8-11.

Craven, R. (1986). Teach the elderly to prevent falls. *Journal of Gerontological Nursing, 12*(8), 27-33.

Cwikel, J., Kaplan, G., & Barell, V. (1990). Falls and subjective health rating among the elderly: Evidence from two Israeli samples. *Social Science Medicine, 31,* 485-490.

Daleiden, S. (1990). Prevention of falling: Rehabilitative or compensatory interventions? *Topics in Geriatric Rehabilitation, 5*(2), 44-53.

Dallaire, L. B., & Burke, E. V. (1989). A new program for reducing patient falls. *Nursing, 19*(1), 65.

Davie, J., Blumenthal, M., & Robinson-Hewlens, S. (1981). A model of risk of falling for psychogeriatric patients. *Archives of Geriatric Psychiatry, 38,* 463-467.

Davis, P. (1981). Human factors contributing to slips, trips and falls. *Ergonomics, 1,* 51-59.

Easterling, M. L. (1990). Which of your patients is headed for a fall? *RN, 53*(1), 56-59.

Edelstein, R., & Merrill, R. (1983). *Falls: A new solution for an old problem.* Unpublished manuscript.

Elnicki, R. A., & Schmitt, J. P. (1980). Contribution of patient and hospital characteristics to adverse patient incidents. *Health Services Research, 15,* 397-414.

English, R. A. (1986). Facing the future: One hospital's approach to nursing the elderly. *Canadian Nurse, 82,* 31-33.

Fagerhaugh, S., Strauss, A., Suczek, B., & Wiener, C. (1980). The impact of technology on patients, providers, and care patterns. *Nursing Outlook, 28,* 666-672.

Feist, R. (1978). A survey of accidental falls in a small home for the aged. *Journal of Gerontological Nursing, 6,* 15-17.

Fife, D., Solomon, P., & Stanton, M. (1984). A risk/falls program: Code orange for success. *Nursing Management, 15*(11), 50-53.

Fine, W. (1959). An analysis of 277 falls in hospitals. *Gerontological Clinics, 1,* 292-300.

Foerster, J. (1981). A study of falls: The elderly nursing home resident. *Journal of the New York State Nursing Association, 2,* 9-17.

Gabell, A., Simons, M. A., & Nayak, U. S. L. (1985). Falls in the healthy elderly: predisposing causes. *Ergonomics, 28,* 965-975.

Gates, S. J. (1984). Helping your patient on bedrest cope with perceptual/sensory deprivation. *Orthopaedic Nursing, 3*(2), 35-38.

Hendrich, A. L. (1988). Unit based fall prevention. *Journal of Quality Assurance, 10*(1), 15-17.

Hernandez, M., & Miller, J. (1986). How to reduce falls. *Geriatric Nursing, 7,* 97-102.

Hibbs, P. J. (1992). Risks, dignity & responsibility in residential homes for the elderly: Freedom or restraint. *Journal of Royal Society of Health, 112,* 199-201.

High quality long-term care for elderly people. (1992). *Journal of the Royal College of Physicians of London, 26,* 130-133.

Hill, B. A., Johnson, R., & Garrett, B. J. (1988). Reducing the incidence of falls in high risk patients. *Journal of Nursing Administration, 18*(7, 8), 24-28.

Hogue, C. (1982). Injury in late life: II. Prevention. *Journal of the American Gerontological Association, 30,* 276-280.

Innes, E. (1985). Maintaining fall prevention. *Quality Review Bulletin, 11,* 217-221.

Innes, E., & Turman, W. (1983). Evaluation of patient falls. *Quality Review Bulletin, 9*(2), 30-45.

James, B. (1983). Accident prevention—establish safety program. *Dimensions in Health Service, 60*(5), 21.

Janken, J., Reynolds, B., & Swiech, K. (1986). Patient falls in the acute care setting: Identifying risk factors. *Nursing Research, 35,* 215-219.

Kalchthaler, T., Bascon, R., & Quintos, U. (1978). Falls in the institutionalized elderly. *Journal of the American Geriatric Society, 26,* 424-428.

Kostopoulos, M. (1985). Reducing patient falls. *Orthopedic Nursing, 4*(6), 14-15.

Kulikowski, E. (1979). A study of accidents in a hospital. *Supervisory Nurse, 10,* 44-45.

Kustaborder, M. (1983). Interventions for safety. *Journal of Gerontological Nursing, 9*(3), 159-162, 173, 182.

Lawrence, J. I., & Maher, P. L. (1992). An interdisciplinary falls consult team: A collaborative approach to patient falls. *Journal of Nursing Care Quality, 6*(3), 21-29.

Lichtenstein, M. J. (1992). Hearing and visual impairments. *Clinics in Geriatric Medicine, 8*(1), 173-182.

Llewellyn, J., Martin, B., Shekleton, M., & Firlit, S. (1988). Analysis of falls in the acute surgical and cardiovascular surgical patient. *Applied Nursing Research, 1*(3), 116-121.

Louis, M. (1983). Falls and causes. *Journal of Gerontological Nursing, 3,* 143-149, 156.

Lund, C., & Sheafor, M. (1985). Is your patient about to fall? *Journal of Gerontological Nursing, 4,* 37-41.

Lynn, I. (1980). Incidents—need they be accidents? *American Journal of Nursing, 80,* 1098-1101.

Maciorowski, L. F., Munro, B. H., Dietrick-Gallagher, M., McNew, C. D., Sheppard-Hinkel, E., Wanich, C., & Ragan, P. A. (1988). A review of the patient fall literature. *Journal of Nursing Quality Assurance, 3*(1), 18-27.

Mayo, N. E., Korner-Bitensky, N., Becker, R., & Georges, P. C. (1989). Preventing falls among patients in a rehabilitation hospital. *Canadian Journal of Rehabilitation, 222,* 235-240.

Morgan, V. R., Mathison, J. H., Rice, J. C., & Clemmer, D. I. (1985). Hospital falls: A persistent problem. *American Journal of Public Health, 75,* 775-777.

Morse, J. M. (1986). Computerized evaluation of a scale to identify the fall-prone patient. *Canadian Journal of Public Health, 77*(Suppl. 1), 21-25.

Morse, J. M., Tylko, S. J., & Dixon, H. A. (1985). The patient who falls . . . and falls again: Defining the aged at risk. *Journal of Gerontological Nursing, 11*(11), 15-18.

Morse, J. M., Tylko, S. J., & Dixon, H. A. (1987). Characteristics of the fall-prone patient. *The Gerontologist, 27,* 516-522.

Patel, K. P. (1976). Falls and faints in the elderly: Look to their clinical history for clues. *Modern Geriatrics, 6,* 28-34.

Regensburg, L. (1988). Falls in the elderly. *Nursing RSA Verpleging, 3,* 24-27.

Riffle, K. L. (1982). Falls: Kinds, causes and prevention. *Geriatric Nursing, 3,* 165-169.

Robbins, A. S., Rubenstein, L. Z., Josephson, M. P. H., Shulman, B. L., Osterweil, D., & Fine, G. (1989). Predictors of falls among elderly people: Results from two population-based studies. *Internal Medicine, 149,* 1628-1633.

Rohde, J. M., Myers, A. H., & Vlahov, D. (1990). Variation in risk for falls by clinical department: Implications for prevention. *Infection Control and Hospital Epidemiology, 11,* 521-524.

Ross, J. E. R. (1991). Iatrogenesis in the elderly: Contributors to falls. *Journal of Gerontological Nursing, 17*(9), 19-23.

Rousseau, P. C. (1985). Falls in the elderly. *Postgraduate Medicine, 78*(6), 87-88.

Rubenstein, L. Z. (1983). Falls in the elderly: A clinical approach. *Western Journal of Medicine, 138,* 273-275.

Rubenstein, L. Z., & Robbins, A. S. (1989). Falling syndromes in elderly persons. *Comprehensive Therapy, 15*(6), 13-18.

Sewell, J. M. A., Spooner, L. L. R., Dixon, A. K., & Rubenstein, D. (1981). Screening investigations in the elderly. *Age and Ageing, 10,* 165-168.

Smith, C. (1976). Accidents and the elderly. *Nursing Times, 72,* 1872-1874.

Spellbring, A. M. (1992). Assessing elderly patients at high risk for falls: A reliability study. *Journal of Nursing Care Quality, 6*(3), 30-35.

Spellbring, A. M., Gannon, M. E., Kleckner, T., & Conway, K. (1988). Improving safety for hospitalized elderly. *Journal of Gerontological Nursing, 14*(2), 31-37.

Spilker, J. A., & Semonin-Holleran, R. (1987). Injury, potential for, related to sensory or motor deficits: Using the stroke scale to validate defining characteristics of this nursing diagnosis. In A. McLane (Ed.), *Classification of nursing diagnoses: Proceedings of the seventh conference* (pp. 247-252). St. Louis, MO: C. V. Mosby.

Stegman, M. R. (1983). Falls among elderly hypertensives—are they iatrogenic? *Gerontology, 29,* 399-406.

Sumner, E. D., & Simpson, W. J. (1992). Intervention in falls among the elderly. *Journal of Practical Nursing, 42*(2), 24-34.

Tideiksaar, R., & Kay, A. (1986). What causes falls? A logical diagnostic procedure. *Geriatrics, 41*(12), 32-44, 47-50.

Tieaskiel, L. (1989). Preventing falls. *Journal of Practical Nursing, 39*(4), 32-35.

Tinetti, M. E., Williams, T. F., & Mayewski, R. (1986). Fall risk index for elderly patients based on number of chronic disabilities. *American Journal of Medicine, 80,* 429-434.

Tisserand, M. (1985). Progress in the prevention of falls caused by slipping. *Ergonomics, 28,* 1027-1042.

Tobis, J. S., Block, M., Steinhaus-Donham, C., Reinsch, S., & Tamaru, K. (1990). Falling among the sensorially impaired elderly. *Archives of Physical Medicine and Rehabilitation, 71,* 144-147.

Venglarik, J. M., & Adams, M. (1985). Which client is a high risk? *Journal of Gerontological Nursing, 11*(5), 28-30.

Walshe, A., & Rosen, H. (1979). A study of patient falls from bed. *Journal of Nursing Administration, 79,* 31-35.

Warshaw, G. A., Moore, J. T., Friedman, W. S., Currie, C. T., Kennie, D. C., Kane, W. J., & Mears, P. A. (1982). Functional disability in the hospitalized elderly. *Journal of the American Medical Association, 248,* 847-850.

Way, B. B. (1992). The relationship between staff-patient ratio and reported patient incidents. *Hospital and Community Psychiatry, 43,* 361-365.

Whedon, M. B., & Shedd, P. (1989). Prediction and prevention of patient falls. *Image: Journal of Nursing Scholarship, 21*(2), 108-114.

Whipple, R. H., Wolfson, L. I., & Amerman, P. M. (1987). The relationship of knee and ankle weakness to falls in nursing home residents: An isokinetic study. *Journal of the American Geriatrics Society, 35*(1), 13-20.

Winograd, C. H. (1991). Targeting strategies: An overview of criteria and outcomes. *Journal of the American Geriatrics Society, 39,* 25S-35S.

Woollacott, M. H. (1990). Changes in posture and voluntary control in the elderly: Research findings and rehabilitation. *Topics in Geriatric Rehabilitation, 5*(2), 1-11.

Wootton, R., Bryson, E., Elsasser, U., Freeman, H., Green, J. R., Hesp, R., Hudson, E. A., Klenerman, L., Smith, T., & Zanelli, J. (1982). Risk factors for fractured neck of femur in the elderly. *Age and Ageing, 11,* 100-107.

Gait Assessment

Alexander, N. B. (1994). Postural control in older adults. *Journal of the American Geriatrics Society, 42,* 93-108.

Chandler, J. M., Duncan, P. W., & Studenski, S. A. (1990). Balance performance on the postural stress test: Comparison of young adults, healthy elderly, and fallers. *Physical Therapy, 70*(7), 410-415.

Crilly, R. G., Willems, D. A., Trenholm, K. J., Hayes, K. C., & Delaquerriere-Richardson, L. F. O. (1989). Effect of exercise on postural sway in the elderly. *Gerontology, 35,* 137-143.

Feltner, M. E., MacRae, P. G., & McNitt-Gray, J. L. (1994). Quantitative gait assessment as a predictor of prospective and retrospective falls in community-dwelling older women. *Archives of Physical Medical Rehabilitation, 75,* 447-453.

Fernie, G. R., Gryfe, C. I., Holliday, P. J., & Llewellyn, A. (1982). The relationship of postural sway in standing to the incidence of falls in geriatric subjects. *Age and Ageing, 11,* 11-16.

Fine, W. (1972). Geriatric ergonomics. *Gerontological Clinics, 14,* 322-332.

Lipsitz, L. A., Nakajima, I., Gagnon, M., Hirayama, T., Connelly, C. M., Izumo, H., & Hirayama, T. (1994). Muscle strength and fall rates among residents of Japanese and American nursing homes: An international cross-cultural study. *Journal of the American Geriatrics Society, 42,* 953-959.

Murphy, J., & Isaacs, B. (1982). The post-fall syndrome. *Gerontology, 28,* 265-270.

Nelson, R. C. (1990). Falls in the elderly. *Emergency Medicine Clinics of North America, 8*(2), 309, 325.

Peszczynski, M. (1965). Why old people fall. *American Journal of Nursing, 5,* 86-88.

Ring, C., Nayak, U. S. L., & Isaacs, B. (1988). Balance function in elderly people who have and who have not fallen. *Archives of Physical Medicine and Rehabilitation, 69,* 261-264.

Sabin, T. D. (1982). Biologic aspects of falls and mobility limitations in the elderly. *Journal of the American Gerontological Association, 30*(1), 51-58.

Scheibel, A. B. (1985). Falls, motor dysfunction, and correlative neurohistologic changes in the elderly. *Clinics in Geriatric Medicine 1,* 671-677.

Stelmach, G. E., & Warringham, C. J. (1985). Sensorimotor deficits related to postural stability: Implications for falling in the elderly. *Clinics in Geriatric Medicine, 1,* 679-694.

Stout, R. W. (1978). Falls and disorders of postural balance. *Age and Ageing, 7*(Suppl.), 134-136.

Tinetti, M. E. (1989). Instability and falling in elderly patients. *Seminars in Neurology, 9*(10), 39-45.

Wolfson, L., Whipple, R., Amerman, P., Kaplan, J., & Kleinberg, A. (1985). Gait and balance in the elderly: Two functional capacities that link sensory and motor ability to falls. *Clinics in Geriatric Medicine, 3,* 649-659.

Wolfson, L., Whipple, R., Amerman, P., & Tobin, J. N. (1990). Gait assessment in the elderly: A gait abnormality rating scale and its relation to falls. *Journal of Gerontology, 45*(1), M12-M19.

Assessment Forms

Berryman, E., Gaskin, D., Jones, A., Tolley, F., & MacMullen, J. (1989). Point by point: Predicting elders' falls. *Geriatric Nursing, 10,* 199-201.

Brians, L. K., Alexander, K., Grota, P., Chen, R. W. H., & Dumas, V. (1991). The development of the RISK tool for fall prevention. *Rehabilitation Nursing, 16*(2), 67-69.

Burden, B., & Kishi, D. (1989). Patient falls: Lowering the risk. *Nursing, 19*(4), 79.

Hendrich, A. L. (1988). An effective unit-based fall prevention plan. *Journal of Nursing Quality Assurance, 3*(1), 28-36.

Hill, B. A., Johnson, R., & Garrett, B. J. (1988). Reducing the incidence of falls in high risk patients. *Journal of Nursing Administration, 18*(7, 8), 24-28.

Morse, J. M., Morse, R. M., & Tylko, S. (1989). Development of a scale to identify the fall-prone patient. *Canadian Journal on Aging, 8,* 366-377.

Rainville, N. (1984). Effect of an implemented fall prevention program. *Quality Review Bulletin, 9,* 287-291.

Ruckstuhl, M. C., Marchionda, E. E., Salmons, J., & Larrabee, J. H. (1991). Patient falls: An outcome indicator. *Journal of Nursing Care Quality, 6*(1), 25-29.

Tideiksaar, R. (1984). An assessment form for falls. *Journal of the American Geriatrics Society, 32,* 538-539.
Tideiksaar, R. (1989). Geriatric falls: Assessing the cause, prevention, preventing recurrence. *Geriatrics, 44*(7), 57-62.
Whedon, M. B., & Shedd, P. (1989). Prediction and prevention of patient falls. *Image: Journal of Nursing Scholarship, 21,* 108-114.

Multidisciplinary Teams

Lawrence, J. I., & Maher, P. L. (1992). An interdisciplinary falls consult team: A collaborative approach to patient falls. *Journal of Nursing Care Quality, 6*(3), 21-29.

Medications

Brown, B. (1983). Study of patient falls in a small, busy medical center. *Critical Care Update, 8,* 30-36.
Campbell, J. A. (1991). Drug treatment as a cause of falls in old age. *Drugs & Aging, 1,* 289-302.
Cumming, R. G., Miller, J. P., Kelsey, J. L., Davis, P., Arfken, C. L., Birge, S. J., & Peck, W. A. (1991). Medications and multiple falls in elderly people: The St. Louis OASIS Study. *Age and Ageing, 20,* 455-461.
Granek, E., Baker, S. P., Abbey, H., Robinson, E., Myers, A. H., Samkoff, J. S., & Klein, L. E. (1987). Medications and diagnoses in relation to falls in a long-term care facility. *Journal of the American Geriatrics Society, 35,* 503-511.
Ladimer, I. (1975). Accidents in the aged: Medicolegal implications. *New York State Journal of Medicine, 14,* 381-387.
Macdonald, J. (1985). The role of drugs in falls in the elderly. *Clinics in Geriatric Medicine, 1,* 621-636.
Macdonald, J., & MacDonald, E. (1977). Nocturnal femoral fracture and continuing widespread use of barbiturates hypnotics. *British Medical Journal, 2,* 483-485.
Ray, W. A., & Griffin, M. R. (1990). Prescribed medications and the risk of falling. *Topics in Geriatric Medicine, 5*(2), 12-20.
Schoenberger, J. A. (1991). Drug-induced orthostatic hypotension. *Drug Safety, 6,* 402-407.
Sobel, K. G., & McCart, G. M. (1983). Drug use and accidental falls in an intermediate care facility. *Drug Intelligence and Clinical Pharmacy, 17,* 539-542.
Stolley, J. M., Buckwalter, K. C., Fjordbak, B., & Bush, S. (1991). Iatrogenesis in the elderly: Drug related problems. *Journal of Gerontological Nursing, 17*(9), 12-17.
Wells, B. G., Middleton, B., Lawrence, G., Lillard, D., & Safarik, J. (1985). Factors associated with the elderly falling in intermediate care facilities. *Drug Intelligence and Clinical Pharmacy, 19,* 142-145.

Yip, Y. B., & Cumming, R. G. (1994). The association between medications and falls in Australian nursing-home residents. *Medical Journal of Australia, 160,* 14-18.

Development and Testing of the Morse Fall Scale

McCollam, M. E. (1995). Evaluation and implementation of a research-based falls assessment innovation. *Nursing Clinics of North America, 30,* 507-514.

Morse, J. M. (1986). Computerized evaluation of a scale to identify the fall-prone patient. *Canadian Journal of Public Health, 77*(Suppl. 1), 21-25.

Morse, J. M. (1994). Strategies for preventing resident falls. *PADONA/LTC, 7*(1), 15-22. Reprinted in *ASLTCN (American Society for Long Term Care) Journal, 5*(1), 15-22.

Morse, J. M., & McHutchion, E. (1991). Releasing restraints: Providing safe care for the elderly. *Research in Nursing & Health, 14,* 187-196.

Morse, J. M., & Morse, R. M. (1988). Calculating fall rates: Methodological concerns. *Quality Review Bulletin, 14*(12), 369-371.

Morse, J. M., Morse, R. M., & Tylko, S. J. (1989). Development of a scale to identify the fall-prone patient. *Canadian Journal on Aging, 8,* 366-377.

Morse, J. M., Prowse, M. D., Morrow, N., & Federspeil, G. (1985). A retrospective analysis of patient falls. *Canadian Journal of Public Health, 76,* 116-118.

Morse, J. M., & Tylko, S. (1985). The use of qualitative methods in a study examining patient falls. In *Human problems: The health context.* Symposium conducted at the meeting of the Nursing and Anthropology Society for Applied Anthropology, Washington, DC.

Morse, J. M., Tylko, S. J., & Dixon, H. A. (1985). The patient who falls . . . and falls again: Defining the aged at risk. *Journal of Gerontological Nursing, 11*(11), 15-18.

Morse, J. M., Tylko, S. J., & Dixon, H. A. (1987). Characteristics of the fall-prone patient. *The Gerontologist, 27,* 516-522.

Environmental Protection

Archea, J. (1985). Environmental factors associated with stair accidents by the elderly. *Clinics in Geriatric Medicine, 3,* 555-569.

Connell, B. R. (1988). Opportunities for environment and behavior research on falls among the elderly. *Environmental Design Research Association, 19,* 223-229.

Cutson, T. M. (1994). Falls in the elderly. *American Family Physician, 49,* 149-156.

Fitzsimons, V. M. (1985). Maintaining a positive environment for the older adult. *Orthopedic Nursing, 4*(3), 48-51.

Healey, F. (1994). Does flooring type affect risk of injury in older in-patients? *Nursing Times, 90*(27), 40-41.

Holliday, P., Fernie, G., & Lauzon, F. (1985). Some bio-engineering approaches to the falling problem. *Geriatric Medicine, 1,* 161-164.

Kolanowski, A. M. (1992). The clinical importance of environmental lighting to the elderly. *Journal of Gerontological Nursing, 18*(1), 10-14.

Maki, B. E., Bartlett, S. A., & Fernie, G. R. (1984). Influence of stairway handrail height on the ability to generate stabilizing forces and moments. *Human Factors, 26,* 704-714.

Maki, B. E., Bartlett, S. A., & Fernie, G. R. (1985). Effect of stairway pitch on optimal handrail height. *Human Factors, 27,* 355-350.

Maxwell, R. J., Bader, J. E., & Watson, W. H. (1972). Territory and self in a geriatric setting. *The Gerontologist, 12,* 413-417.

Miller, J. (1989). Practical tips on reducing hazards of falls [Letter to the editor]. *American Journal of Public Health, 79,* 1056.

Owen, D. H. (1985). Maintaining posture and avoiding tripping: Optical information for detecting and controlling orientation and locomotion. *Clinics in Geriatric Medicine, 3,* 581-599.

Tideiksaar, R. (1990). Environment adaptations to preserve balance and prevent falls. *Topics in Geriatric Rehabilitation, 5*(2), 78-86.

Waller, J. A. (1978). Falls among the elderly—human and environmental factors. *Accident Annals and Preventions, 10,* 21-33.

Wong, S., Glennie, K., Muise, M., Lambie, E., & Meagher, D. (1981). An exploration of environmental variables and patient falls. *Dimensions in Health Services, 58,* 9-11.

Fall Prevention Programs

Cohen, L., & Guin, P. (1991). Implementation of a patient fall prevention program. *Journal of Neuroscience Nursing, 23,* 315-319.

Halpert, A., & Connors, J. P. (1986). Prevention of patient falls through perceived control and other techniques. *Law, Medicine & Health Care, 14*(1), 20-24.

Harris, P. B. (1989). Organizational and staff attitudinal determinants of falls in nursing home residents. *Medical Care, 27,* 737-749.

Hart, M. A., & Sliefert, M. K. (1983). Monitoring patient incidents in a long term care facility. *Quality Review Bulletin, 9,* 356-365.

Kilpack, V. (1991). Using research-based interventions to decrease patient falls. *Applied Nursing Research, 4*(2), 50-56.

Kustaborder, M. (1983). Interventions for safety. *Journal of Gerontological Nursing, 9*(3), 159-162, 173, 182.

Morse, J. M. (1994). Strategies for preventing resident falls. *PADONA/LTC, 7*(1), 15-22. Reprinted in *ASLTCN (American Society for Long Term Care) Journal, 5*(1), 15-22.

Ruckstuhl, M. C., Marchionda, E. E., Salmons, J., & Larrabee, J. H. (1991). Patient falls: An outcome indicator. *Journal of Nursing Care Quality, 6*(1), 25-29.

Schmid, N. A. (1990). Reducing patient falls: A research-based comprehensive fall prevention program. *Military Medicine, 155,* 202-207.

Tinetti, M. E., Baker, D. I., McAvay, G., Claus, E. B., Garrett, P., Gottschalk, M., Koch, M. L., Trainor, K., & Horwitz, R. I. (1994). A multifactorial intervention to reduce the risk of falling among elderly people living in the community. *New England Journal of Medicine, 331,* 821-827.

Tutuarima, J. A., de Haan, R. J., & Limburg, M. (1993). Number of nursing staff and falls: A case-control study on falls by stroke patients in acute-care settings. *Journal of Advanced Nursing, 18,* 1101-1105.

Fall Rates

Berry, G., Fisher, R., & Lang, S. (1981). Detrimental incidents including falls in an elderly institutionalized population. *Journal of the American Gerontological Association, 29,* 322-324.

Bronstein, J., & Zalar, M. (1983). *Reduce the incidence of patient falls in an acute care setting.* Unpublished manuscript.

Buehrle, R. (1969). When where how and why of accidents among patients. *Hospital Administration in Canada, 11*(12), 24-28.

Campbell, A., Reinken, J., Allan, B., & Martinez, G. (1981). Falls in old age: A study of frequency and related clinical factors. *Age and Ageing, 10,* 264-270.

Daley, I., & Goldman, L. (1987). A closer look at institutional accidents. *Geriatric Nursing, 8*(2), 64-67.

Duthie, E. H., & Gambert, S. R. (1983). Accident and fall prevention in the elderly. *Wisconsin Medical Journal, 82*(9), 23-25.

Eddy, T. (1973). Deaths from falls and fractures: Comparison of mortality in Scotland and the United States with that of England and Wales. *British Journal of Preventive Medicine, 27,* 247-254.

Elliott, D. F. (1979). Accidents in nursing homes: Implications for patients and administrators. In M. B. Miller (Ed.), *Current issues in clinical geriatrics* (pp. 97-134). New York: Tiresias.

Fagin, I. D. (1965). Who? Where? When? How? An analysis of 868 inpatient accidents. *Hospitals, J.A.H.A., 39,* 60-64.

Gibbs, J. (1982). Bed area falls: A recent report. *Australian Nurses Journal, 11,* 34-37.

Grant, J., & Hamilton, S. (1987). Falls in a rehabilitation center: A retrospective and comparative analysis. *Rehabilitation Nursing, 12*(2), 74-76.

Gryfe, C., Amies, A., & Ashley, M. (1977). A longitudinal study of falls in an elderly population: I. Incidence and morbidity. *Age and Ageing, 6,* 201-210.

Gurwitz, J. H., Sanchez-Cross, M. T., Eckler, M. A., & Matulis, J. (1994). The epidemiology of adverse and unexpected events in the long-term care setting. *Journal of the American Geriatrics Society, 42,* 33-38.

Hogue, C. C. (1980). Injury in late life, Part 1: Epidemiology of injury in older age. *Journal of the American Geriatrics Society, 30,* 183-190.

Hogue, C. C. (1977). Epidemiology of injury in older age. In S. G. Haynes (Ed.), *Proceedings of the Second Conference on the Epidemiology of Aging, March 28-29, 1977* (pp. 127-138). Bethesda, MD: National Institutes of Health.

Jèrvinen, K., & Jèrvinen, P. (1968). Falling from bed as a complication of hospital treatment. *Journal of Chronic Disease, 21,* 375-378.

Johnson, E. (1985). Accidental falls among geriatric patients: Can more be prevented? *Journal of the National Medical Association, 77,* 633-639.

Jones, W. J., & Smith, A. (1989). Preventing hospital incidents—what can we do? *Nursing Management, 20*(9), 58-60.

Le Bourdais, E. (1977). A Canadian survey: Accidents in hospitals. *Dimensions in Health Services, 54*(2), 25-28.

Llewellyn, J., Martin, B., Shekleton, M., & Firlit, S. (1988). Analysis of falls in the acute surgical and cardiovascular surgical patient. *Applied Nursing Research, 1*(3), 116-121.

Lucht, U. (1971). A prospective study of accidental falls and resulting injuries in the home among elderly people. *Acta Socio-medica Scandinavica, 2,* 105-120.

Manjam, N. V. B., & MacKinnon, H. H. (1973). Patient, bed and bathroom: A study of falls occurring in a general hospital. *Nova Scotia Medical Bulletin, 52,* 23-25.

Manning, D. P. (1983). Deaths and injuries caused by slipping, tripping and falling. *Ergonomics, 26*(1), 3-9.

Margulec, I., Librach, G., & Schadel, M. (1970). Epidemiological study of accidents among residents of homes for the aged. *Journal of Gerontology, 25,* 342-346.

Miceli, D. L. G., Wasman, H., Cavalieri, T., & Lage, S. (1994). Prodromal falls among older nursing home residents. *Applied Nursing Research, 7*(1), 18-27.

Mion, L. C., Gregor, S., Buettner, M., Chwirchak, D., Lee, O., & Paras, W. (1989). Falls in the rehabilitation setting: Incidence and characteristics. *Rehabilitation Nursing, 14*(1), 17-21.

Mitchell, R. G. (1984). Falls in the elderly. *Nursing Times, 80*(2), 51-53.

Moorat, D. (1983). Accidents to patients. *Nursing Times, 79*(20), 59-61.

Morgan, V. R., Mathison, J. H., Rice, J. C., & Clemmer, D. I. (1985). Hospital falls: A persistent problem. *American Journal of Public Health, 75,* 775-777.

Morris, E. V., & Isaacs, B. (1980). The prevention of falls in geriatric hospital. *Age and Ageing, 9,* 181-185.

Morse, J. M., Prowse, M. D., Morrow, N., & Federspeil, G. (1985). A retrospective analysis of patient falls. *Canadian Journal of Public Health, 76,* 116-118.

Overstall, P. W. (1978). Falls in the elderly—epidemiology, etiology and management. In B. Isaacs (Ed.), *Recent advances in geriatric medicine* (pp. 61-72). New York: Churchill-Livingstone.

Overstall, P. W., Johnson, A. L., & Exton-Smith, A. N. (1978). Instability and falls in the elderly. *Age and Ageing, 7*(Suppl.), 92-96.

Pablo, R. Y. (1977). Patient accidents in a long-term care facility. *Canadian Journal of Public Health, 68,* 237-247.

Parrish, H. M., & Weil, T. P. (1958). Patient accidents occurring in hospitals: Epidemiologic study of 614 accidents. *New York State Journal of Medicine, 58,* 838-840.

Perry, B. C. (1982). Falls among the elderly: A review of the methods and conclusions of epidemiologic studies. *Journal of the American Gerontological Association, 30,* 367-372.

Raz, T., & Baretich, M. F. (1987). Factors affecting the incidence of patient falls in hospitals. *Medical Care, 25*(3), 185-195.

Ross, J. E. R. (1991). Iatrogenesis in the elderly. *Journal of Gerontological Nursing, 17*(9), 19-23.

Scott, C. J. (1976). Accidents in hospital with special reference to old people. *Health Bulletin, 34,* 330-335.

Sehested, P., & Severin-Nielsen, T. (1977). Falls by hospitalized elderly patients: Causes, prevention. *Geriatrics, 32*(4), 101-108.

Sheldon, J. H. (1960). On the natural history of falls in old age. *British Medical Journal, 2*(5214), 1685-1690.

Sorock, G. S. (1983). A case control study of falling incidents among the hospitalized elderly. *Journal of Safety Research, 14,* 47-52.

Spasoff, R. A., Kraus, A. S., Beattie, E. J., Holden, D. E. W., Lawson, J. S., Rodenburg, M., & Woodcock, G. M. (1978). A longitudinal study of elderly residents of long-stay institutions. *The Gerontologist, 18,* 281-292.

Stone, E. P. (1962). What is a reasonable "standard rate" for patient accidents? *Journal of the American Hospitals Association, Part 2,* 43-46, 114.

Swartzbeck, E. M. (1983). The problems of falls in the elderly. *Nursing Management, 14*(2), 34-38.

Swartzbeck, E. M., & Milligan, W. C. (1982). A comparative study of hospital incidents. *Nursing Management, 13*(1), 39-43.

Tinker, G. M. (1979). Accidents in a geriatric department. *Age and Ageing, 8,* 196-198.

Uden, G. (1985). Inpatient accidents in hospitals. *Journal of the American Geriatrics Society, 33,* 833-841.

Vlahov, D., Myers, A. H., & Al-Ibrahim, M. S. (1990). Epidemiology of falls among patients in a rehabilitation hospital. *Archives of Physical Medicine and Rehabilitation, 71,* 8-12.

Walsh, J. B. (1989). To trip, to slip, perchance to tumble. *Irish Medical Journal, 82*(2), 52-53.

Winter, D. A., Patla, A. E., Frank, J. S., & Walt, S. E. (1990). Biomechanical walking pattern changes in the fit and healthy elderly. *Physical Therapy, 70,* 340-347.

Falls in the Home and Community

Agate, J. (1966). Accidents to old people in their homes. *British Medical Journal, 2,* 785-788.

Campbell, A. J., Borrie, J. J., & Spears, G. F. (1989). Risk factors for falls in a community-based prospective study of people 70 years and older. *Journal of Gerontology, 44*(4), M112-M117.

Colling, J., & Park, D. (1983). Home, safe home. *Journal of Gerontological Nursing, 9*(3), 175-179, 192.

Downton, J. H., & Andrews, K. (1991). Prevalence, characteristics and factors associated with falls among the elderly living at home. *Aging, 3,* 219-228.

Dunn, J. E., Rudberg, M. A., Furner, S. E., & Cassel, C. (1992). Mortality, disability, and falls in older persons: The role of underlying disease and disability. *American Journal of Public Health, 82,* 395-400.

Gray-Vickrey, M. (1984). Education to prevent falls. *Geriatric Nursing, 5*(3), 179-183.

Hopkins, T. (1988). Heading for a fall. *Geriatric Nursing and Home Care, 7*(8), 10-11.

Moller, J. (1986). Towards injury reduction: The role of hospital based surveillance systems. *Community Health Studies, 10*(2), 161-165.

Morfitt, J. M. (1979). Accidents to old people in residential homes. *Public Health, 93,* 177-184.

Myers, A. H., Baker, S. P., Robinson, E. G., Abbey, H., Doll, E. T., & Levenson, S. (1989). Falls in the institutionalized elderly. *Journal of Long-Term Care Administration, 17*(4), 12-18.

Nickens, H. (1985). Intrinsic factors in falling among the elderly. *Archives of Internal Medicine, 145,* 1089-1093.

Prudham, D., & Evans, J. G. (1981). Factors associated with falls in the elderly: A community study. *Age and Ageing, 10,* 141-146.

Tinetti, M. E. (1988). Risk factors for falls among elderly persons living in the community. *New England Journal of Medicine, 319*(26), 1701-1707.

Wild, D., Nayak, U. S. L., & Isaacs, B. (1981). How dangerous are falls in old people at home? *British Medical Journal, 282*(6260), 266-268.

Witte, S. N. (1979). Why the elderly fall. *American Journal of Nursing, 79,* 1950-1952.

Injuries and Outcomes of Falls

Baker, S., & Harvey, A. H. (1985). Fall injuries in the elderly. *Clinics in Geriatric Medicine, 1,* 501-512.

Brocklehurst, J. C., Exton-Smith, A. N., Lempert Barber, S. M., Hunt, L. P., & Palmer, M. K. (1978). Fracture of the femur in old age: A two-centre study of associated clinical factors and the cause of the fall. *Age and Ageing, 7*(7), 2-15.

Chipman, C., & Sarant, G. (1981). What does it mean when a patient falls? Part II. *Geriatrics, 36*(10), 101-105.

Clark, G. (1985). A study of falls among elderly hospitalized patients. *Australian Journal of Advanced Nursing, 2*(2), 34-44.

Dimant, J. (1985). Accidents in the skilled nursing facility. *New York State Journal of Medicine, 85,* 202-205.

Haga, H., Shibata, H., Shichita, K., Toshihisa, M., & Hatano, S. (1986). Falls in the institutionalized elderly in Japan. *Archives of Gerontological Geriatrics, 5,* 1-9.

Rozycki, G. S., & Maull, K. I. (1991). Injuries sustained by falls. *Archives of Emergency Medicine, 8,* 245-252.

Waller, J. A. (1974). Injury in the aged: Clinical and epidemiological implications. *New York State Journal of Medicine, 74*(12), 2200-2208.

White, L., Farmer, M., & Brody, J. (1984). Who is at risk? Hip fracture epidemiology report. *Journal of Gerontological Nursing, 10*(10), 26-30.

Wild, D., Nayak, U. S. L., & Isaacs, B. (1981). Prognosis of falls in old people at home. *Journal of Epidemiology and Community Health, 35*(3), 200-204.

Prevention Programs

Berryman, E., Gaskin, D., Jones, A., Tolley, F., & MacMullen, J. (1989). Point by point: Predicting elders' falls. *Geriatric Nursing, 10*(4), 199-201.

Fiatarone, M. A., & Evans, W. J. (1990). Exercise in the oldest old. *Topics in Geriatric Rehabilitation, 5*(2), 63-77.

Kilpack, V. (1991). Using research-based interventions to decrease patient falls. *Applied Nursing Research, 4*(2), 50-56.

Lamb, K., Miller, J., & Hernandez, M. (1987). Falls in the elderly: Cause and prevention. *Orthopaedic Nursing, 6*(2), 45-49.

Morse, J. M. (1994). Strategies for preventing resident falls. *PADONA/LTC, 7*(1), 15-22. Reprinted in *ASLTCN (American Society for Long Term Care) Journal, 5*(1), 15-22.

Morse, J. M., Morse, R. M., & Tylko, S. J. (1989). Development of a scale to identify the fall-prone patient. *Canadian Journal on Aging, 8,* 366-377.

Ruckstuhl, M. C., Marchionda, E. E., Salmons, J., & Larrabee, J. H. (1991). Patient falls: An outcome indicator. *Journal of Nursing Care Quality, 6*(1), 25-29.

Whedon, M. B., & Shedd, P. (1989). Prediction and prevention of patient falls. *Image: Journal of Nursing Scholarship, 21*(2), 108-114.

Young, S. W., Abedzadeh, C. H., & White, M. W. (1989). A fall-prevention program for nursing homes. *Nursing Management, 20*(11), 80Y-80FF.

Zepp, S. (1991). Ban "a" fall: A nursing innovation to reducing patient falls. *Kansas Nurse, 66*(7), 13.

Multiple Fallers

Catchen, H. (1983). Repeaters: Inpatient accidents among hospitalized elderly. *The Gerontologist, 23,* 273-276.

Dunn, J. E., Rudberg, M. A., Furner, S. E., & Cassel, C. (1992). Mortality, disability, and falls in older persons: The role of underlying disease and disability. *American Journal of Public Health, 82*(3), 395.

Fiesta, J. (1985). Nursing liability—the patient who falls. *Orthopedic Nursing, 3,* 59-61.

Gross, Y. T., Shimamoto, Y., Rose, C. L., & Frank, B. (1990). Why do they fall? Monitoring risk factors in nursing homes. *Journal of Gerontological Nursing, 16*(6), 20-25.

Livesley, B., & Atkinson, L. (1974). Repeated falls in the elderly. *Modern Geriatrics, 4,* 458-467.

Morse, J. M., Tylko, S. J., & Dixon, H. A. (1985). The patient who falls . . . and falls again: Defining the aged at risk. *Journal of Gerontological Nursing, 11*(11), 15-18.

Wright, B. A., Aizenstein, S., Vogler, G., Rowe, M., & Miller, C. (1990). Frequent fallers: Leading groups to identify psychological factors. *Journal of Gerontological Nursing, 16*(4), 15-19.

Outcomes

Borkan, J. M., Quirk, M., & Sullivan, M. (1991). Finding meaning after the fall: Injury narratives from elderly hip fracture patients. *Social Science & Medicine, 33,* 947-957.

Campbell, E. B., Williams, M. A., & Mlynarczyk, S. M. (1986). After the fall—confusion. *American Journal of Nursing, 86*(2), 151-153.

Franzoni, S., Rozzini, R., Boffelli, S., Frisoni, G. B., & Trabucchi, M. (1994). Fear of falling in nursing home patients. *Gerontology, 40,* 38-44.

Miceli, D. L. G., Wasman, H., Cavalieri, T., & Lage, S. (1994). Prodromal falls among older nursing home residents. *Applied Nursing Research, 7*(1), 18-27.

Morris, J. C., Rubin, E. H., Morris, E. J., & Mandel, S. A. (1987). Senile dementia of the Alzheimer's type: An important risk factor for serious falls. *Journal of Gerontology, 42,* 412-417.

Restraints

Brower, H. T. (1991). The alternatives to restraints. *Journal of Gerontological Nursing, 17*(2), 18-22.

Brungardt, G. S. (1994). Patient restraints: New guidelines for a less restrictive approach. *Geriatrics, 49*(6), 43-50.

Burton, L. C., German, P. S., Rovner, B. W., & Brant, L. J. (1992). Physical restraint use and cognitive decline among nursing home residents. *Journal of the American Geriatrics Society, 40,* 811-816.

Byers, V., Arrington, M. E., & Finstuen, K. (1990). Predictive risk factors associated with stroke patient falls in acute care settings. *Journal of Neuroscience Nursing, 22*(3), 147-154.

Clavon, A. M. (1991). Implementation of a restraint policy: A case study. *Military Medicine, 156,* 499-501.

Cutchins, C. H. (1991). Blueprint for restraint-free care. *American Journal of Nursing, 91*(7), 36-42.

Ejaz, F. K., Jones, J. A., & Rose, M. S. (1994). Falls among nursing home residents: An examination of incident reports before and after restraint reduction programs. *Journal of the American Geriatrics Society, 42,* 960-964.

Folmar, S., & Wilson, H. (1989). Social behavior and physical restraints. *The Gerontologist, 29,* 650-653.

Janelli, L. M., Scherer, Y. K., Kanski, G. W., & Neary, M. A. (1991). What nursing staff members really know about physical restraints. *Rehabilitation Nursing, 16,* 345-349.

Kallmann, S. L. (1992). Comfort, safety, and independence: Restraint release and its challenges. *Geriatric Nursing, 13*(3), 143-148.

Magee, R., Hyatt, E. C., Hardin, S. B., Stratmann, D., Vinson, M. H., & Owen, M. (1993). Institutional policy: Use of restraints in extended care and nursing homes. *Journal of Gerontological Nursing, 19*(4), 31-39.

Marks, W. (1992). Physical restraints in the practice of medicine: Current concepts [Review]. *Archives of Internal Medicine, 152,* 2203-2206.

Masters, R., & Marks, S. F. (1990). The use of restraints. *Rehabilitation Nursing, 15*(1), 22-25.

McHutchion, E., & Morse, J. M. (1990). Releasing restraints: A nursing dilemma. *Journal of Gerontological Nursing, 15*(2), 16-21.

Morse, J. M., & McHutchion, E. (1991). The behavioral effects of releasing restraints. *Research in Nursing and Health, 14,* 187-196.

Morton, D. (1989). Five years of fewer falls. *American Journal of Nursing, 89,* 204-205.

Rader, J. (1991). Modifying the environment to decrease use of restraints. *Journal of Gerontological Nursing, 17*(2), 9-13.

Restraints and bedfalls: Most frequent accidents. (1983). *Regan Report on Nursing Law, 23*(10), 4.

Restraints: Necessity of convenience. (1980). *Proceedings of a workshop of the Ontario Geriatric Association.* Queens Park: Ontario Geriatric Association.

Risk analysis: Physical restraints. (1988, September). *Safety, Security, and Loss Prevention, 6,* 1-6.

Robbins, L. J., Boyko, E., Lane, J., Cooper, D., & Jahnigen, D. W. (1987). Binding the elderly: A prospective study of the use of mechanical restraints in an acute care hospital. *Journal of the American Geriatrics Society, 35,* 290-296.

Schaeffer, J. M., & Miller, H. (1980). Controlling risks in patient transfers. *Hospitals, 54*(14), 46-50.

Spellbring, A. M. (1992). Assessing elderly patients at high risk for falls: A reliability study. *Journal of Nursing Care Quality, 6*(3), 30-35.

Strumpf, N. E., Evans, L. K., & Schwartz, D. (1990). Restraint-free care: From dream to reality. *Geriatric Nursing, 11*(3), 122-124.

Tideiksaar, R. (1989). Restraint use declines as fall prevention options rise. *Provider, 15*(7), 35-36.

Tinetti, M. E., Wen-Liang, L., & Ginter, S. F. (1992). Mechanical restraint use and fall-related injuries among residents of skilled nursing facilities. *Annals of Internal Medicine, 116,* 369-374.

Vellas, B., Cayla, F., Bocquet, H. M., dePemille, F., & Albarede, J. L. (1987). Prospective study of restriction of activity in old people after falls. *Age and Ageing, 16,* 189-193.

Wendkos, M. H. (1980). Psychiatric patients and sudden death [Letter]. *American Journal of Psychiatry, 137,* 1627-1628.

Widder, B. (1985). A new device to decrease falls. *Geriatric Nursing, 6,* 287-288.

Risk Factors

Barbieri, E. G. (1983). Patient falls are not patient accidents. *Journal of Gerontological Nursing, 3,* 165-173.

Greenspan, S. L., Myers, E. R., Maitland, L. A., Resnick, N. M., & Hayes, W. C. (1994). Fall severity and bone mineral density as risk factors for hip fracture in ambulatory elderly. *Journal of the American Medical Association, 271*(2), 128-133.

Lord, S. R., Clark, R. D., & Webster, I. W. (1991). Physiological factors associated with falls in an elderly population. *Journal of the American Geriatrics Society, 39,* 1194-1200.

McVey, L. J., & Studenski, S. A. (1988). Falls in the elderly. In M. G. Eisenberg & R. C. Grzesiak (Eds.), *Advances in clinical rehabilitation* (Vol. 2, pp. 108-131). New York: Springer.

Reporting Falls

Cummings, S. R., Nevitt, M. C., & Kidd, S. (1988). Forgetting falls: The limited accuracy of recall of falls in the elderly. *Journal of the American Geriatrics Society, 36,* 613-616.

Hale, W. A., Delaney, M. J., & Cable, T. (1993). Accuracy of patient recall and chart documentation of falls. *Journal of the American Board of Family Practice, 6,* 239-242.

Mark, B. A., & Burleson, D. L. (1995). Measurement of patient outcomes: Data availability and consistency across hospitals. *Journal of Nursing Administration, 25*(4), 52-59.

References

Apgar, V. (1953). A proposal for a new method of evaluating the newborn infant. *Current Perspectives in Anesthesia and Analgesia, 18,* 260-267.

Arsenault, T. (1982). Slips and falls: Problem identification and resolution by primary nurse. In *Nursing research: Advancing clinical practice for the 80's* (pp. 386-396). Walnut Creek, CA: Symposia Medic.

Baker, S., & Harvey, A. H. (1985). Fall injuries in the elderly. *Clinics in Geriatric Medicine, 3,* 501-512.

Barbieri, E. G. (1983). Patient falls are not patient accidents. *Journal of Gerontological Nursing, 3,* 165-173.

Berry, G., Fisher, R., & Lang, S. (1981). Detrimental incidents including falls in an elderly institutionalized population. *Journal of the American Gerontological Association, 29,* 322-324.

Berryman, E., Gaskin, D., Jones, A., Tolley, F., & MacMullen, J. (1989). Point by point: Predicting elders' falls. *Geriatric Nursing, 10*(4), 199-201.

Brocklehurst, J., Exton-Smith, A., & Barber, S. (1978). Fractures of the femur in old age: A two-centre study of associated clinical factors and the cause of a fall. *Age and Ageing, 11,* 7-15.

Brungardt, G. S. (1994). Patient restraints: New guidelines for a less restrictive approach. *Geriatrics, 49*(6), 43-50.

143

Burton, L. C., German, P. S., Rovner, B. W., & Brant, L. J. (1992). Physical restraint use and cognitive decline among nursing home residents. *Journal of American Geriatric Society, 40,* 811-816.

Campbell, A., Reinken, J., Allan, B., & Martinez, G. (1981). Falls in old age: A study of frequency and related clinical factors. *Age and Ageing, 10,* 264-270.

Catchen, H. (1983). Repeaters: Inpatient accidents among hospitalized elderly. *The Gerontologist, 23,* 273-276.

Cohen, L., & Guin, P. (1991). Implementation of a patient fall prevention program. *Journal of Neuroscience Nursing, 23,* 315-319.

Cohn, T. E., & Lasley, D. (1985). Visual depth illusion and falls in the elderly. *Clinics in Geriatric Medicine, 3,* 601-620.

David, M. A-M. (1987). Report of inquest. Montréal: Le Bureau du Coroner, Gouvernement du. Québec.

Davie, J., Blumenthal, M., & Robinson-Hewlens, S. (1981). A model of risk of falling for psychogeriatric patients. *Archives of Geriatric Psychiatry, 38,* 463-467.

Dawes, R. (1979). The robust beauty of improper linear models in decision making. *American Psychologist, 7,* 571-582.

Ejaz, F. K., Jones, J. A., & Rose, M. S. (1994). Falls among nursing home residents: An examination of incident reports before and after restraint reduction programs. *Journal of the American Geriatrics Society, 42,* 960-964.

Fife, D., Solomon, P., & Stanton, M. (1984). A risk/falls program: Code orange for success. *Nursing Management, 15*(11), 50-53.

Grant, J., & Hamilton, S. (1987). Falls in a rehabilitation center: A retrospective and comparative analysis. *Rehabilitation Nursing, 12*(2), 74-76.

Gryfe, C., Amies, A., & Ashley, M. (1977). A longitudinal study of falls in an elderly population: In incidence and morbidity. *Age and Ageing, 6,* 201-210.

Hendrich, A. L. (1988). An effective unit-based fall prevention plan. *Journal of Nursing Quality Assurance, 3*(1), 28-36.

Holliday, P., Fernie, G., Maki, B. E., & Lauzon, F. (1985). Some bio-engineering approaches to the falling problem. *Geriatric Medicine, 1,* 161-164.

Innes, E., & Turman, W. (1983). Evaluation of patient falls. *Quality Review Bulletin, 2,* 30-45.

Johnson, E. (1985). Accidental falls among geriatric patients: Can more be prevented? *Journal of the National Medical Association, 8,* 633-639.

Kallmann, S. L., Denine-Flynn, M., & Blackburn, D. M. (1992). Comfort, safety, and independence: Restraint release and its challenges. *Geriatric Nursing, 13,* 143-148.

Kilpack, V., Boehm, J., Smith, N., & Mudge, B. (1991). Using research-based interventions to decrease patient falls. *Applied Nursing Research, 4*(2), 50-56.

Lachenbruch, P. (1975). *Discriminate analysis.* New York: Hafner.

Lipsitz, L. (1983). The drop attack: A common geriatric problem. *Journal of American Geriatric Society, 10,* 617-620.

Livesley, B., & Atkinson, L. (1974). Repeated falls in the elderly. *Modern Geriatrics, 4,* 458-467.

Llewellyn, J., Martin, B., Shekleton, M., & Firlit, S. (1988). Analysis of falls in the acute surgical and cardiovascular surgical patient. *Applied Nursing Research, 1*(3), 116-121.

Maki, B. E., Bartlett, S. A., & Fernie, G. R. (1985). Effect of stairway pitch on optimal handrail height. *Human Factors, 27,* 355-350.

McCollam, M. (1995). Evaluation and implementation of a research-based falls assessment innovation. *Nursing Clinics of North America, 30,* 507-514.

Mion, L. C., Gregor, S., Buettner, M., Chwirchak, D., Lee, O., & Paras, W. (1989). Falls in the rehabilitation setting: Incidence and characteristics. *Rehabilitation Nursing, 14,* 17-21.

Morgan, V. R., Mathison, J. H., Rice, J. C., & Clemmer, D. I. (1985). Hospital falls: A persistent problem. *American Journal of Public Health, 75,* 775-777.

Morris, E. V., & Isaacs, B. (1980). The prevention of falls in geriatric hospital. *Age and Ageing, 9,* 1981-1985.

Morris, J. C., Rubin, E. H., Morris, E. J., & Mandel, S. A. (1987). Senile dementia of the Alzheimer's type: An important risk factor for serious falls. *Journal of Gerontology, 42,* 412-417.

Morse, J. M. (1986). Computerized evaluation of a scale to identify the fall prone patient. *Canadian Journal of Public Health, 77* (Suppl. 1), 21-25.

Morse, J. M., Black, C., Oberle, K., & Donahue, P. (1989). A prospective study to identify the fall-prone patient. *Social Science in Medicine, 28*(1), 81-86.

Morse, J. M., & McHutchion, E. (1991). The behavioral effects of releasing restraints. *Research in Nursing and Health, 14,* 187-196.

Morse, J. M., & Morse, R. M. (1988). Calculating fall rates: Methodologic concerns. *Quality Review Bulletin: Journal of Quality Assurance, 14*(12), 369-371.

Morse, J. M., Morse, R. M., & Tylko, S. J. (1989). Development of a scale to identify the fall-prone patient. *Canadian Journal on Aging, 8,* 366-377.

Morse, J. M., Prowse, M. D., Morrow, N., & Federspeil, G. (1985). A retrospective analysis of patient falls. *Canadian Journal of Public Health, 76,* 116-118.

Morse, J. M., Tylko, S. J., & Dixon, H. A. (1985). The patient who falls . . . and falls again: Defining the aged at risk. *Journal of Gerontological Nursing, 11*(11), 15-18.

Morse, J. M., Tylko, S. J., & Dixon, H. A. (1987). Characteristics of the fall-prone patient. *The Gerontologist, 27,* 516-522.

Myers, A. H., Baker, S. P., Robinson, E. G., Abbey, H., Doll, E. T., & Levenson, S. (1989). Falls in the institutionalized elderly. *Journal of Long-Term Care Administration, 17*(4), 12-16.

Overstall, P. W. (1978). Falls in the elderly—Epidemiology, etiology and management. In B. Isaacs (Ed.), *Recent advances in geriatric medicine* (pp. 61-72). New York: Churchill-Livingstone.

Patel, K. P. (1976). Accidents in the home: Falls and faints in the elderly: Look to their clinical history for clues. *Modern Geriatrics, 6,* 28-34.

Rainville, N. (1984). Effect of an implemented fall prevention program. *Quality Review Bulletin, 9,* 287-291.

Raz, T., & Baretich, M. F. (1987). Factors affecting the incidence of patient falls in hospitals. *Medical Care, 25*(3), 185-195.

Restraints: Necessity of convenience. (1980). *Proceedings of a workshop of the Ontario Geriatric Association.* Queens Park: Ontario Geriatric Association.

Robb, S. S., Stegman, C. E., & Wolanin, M. O. (1986). No research versus research with compromised results: A study of validation therapy. *Nursing Research, 35*(2), 113-118.

Ruckstuhl, M. C., Marchionda, E. E., Salmons, J., & Larrabee, J. H. (1991). Patient falls: An outcome indicator. *Journal of Nursing Care Quality, 6*(1), 25-29.

Sehested, P., & Severin-Nielsen, T. (1977). Falls by hospitalized elderly patients: Causes, prevention. *Geriatrics, 4,* 101-108.

Spellbring, A. M., Gannon, M. E., Kleckner, T., & Conway, K. (1988). Improving safety for hospitalized elderly. *Journal of Gerontological Nursing, 14*(2), 31-37.

Strumpf, N. E., Evans, L. K., & Schwartz, D. (1990). Restraint-free care: From dream to reality. *Geriatric Nursing, 11*(3), 122-124.

Tack, K. A., Ulrich, B., & Kehr, C. (1987). Patient falls: Profile for prevention. *Journal of Neuroscience Nursing, 19*(2), 83-89.

Tideiksaar, R. (1984). An assessment form for falls. *Journal of the American Geriatrics Society, 32,* 538-539.

Tideiksaar, R. (1989). Geriatric falls: Assessing the cause, prevention, preventing recurrence. *Geriatrics, 44*(7), 57-62.

Tideiksaar, R., & Kay, A. (1986). What causes falls? A logical diagnostic procedure. *Geriatrics, 41*(12), 42-44, 47-50.

Tinetti, M. E., Williams, T. F., & Mayewski, R. (1986). Fall risk index for elderly patients based on number of chronic disabilities. *American Journal of Medicine, 3,* 429-434.

Tinetti, M. E., Liu, W-L., & Ginter, S. F. (1992). Mechanical restraint use and fall-related injuries among residents of skilled nursing facilities. *Annals of Internal Medicine, 116,* 369-374.

Vlahov, D., Myers, A. H., & Al-Ibrahim, M. S. (1990). Epidemiology of falls among patients in a rehabilitation hospital. *Archives of Physical Medicine and Rehabilitation, 71,* 8-12.

Warshaw, G. A., Moore, J. T., Friedman, W. S., Currie, C. T., Kennie, D. C., Kane, W. J., & Mears, P. A. (1982). Functional disability in the hospitalized elderly. *Journal of the American Medical Association, 248,* 847-850.

Wendkos, M. H. (1980). Psychiatric patients and sudden death [Letter]. *American Journal of Psychiatry, 137,* 1627-1628.

Whedon, M. B., & Shedd, P. (1989). Prediction and prevention of patient falls. *Image: Journal of Nursing Scholarship, 21*(2), 108-114.

Wolfson, L., Whipple, R., Amerman, P., Kaplan, J., & Kleinberg, A. (1985). Gait and balance in the elderly two functional capacities that link sensory and motor ability to falls. *Clinics in Geriatric Medicine, 3,* 649-659.

Wolfson, L., Whipple, R., Amerman, P., & Tobin, J. N. (1990). Gait assessment in the elderly: A gait abnormality rating scale and its relation to falls. *Journal of Gerontology, 45*(1), M12-M19.

Wright, B. A., Aizenstein, S., Vogler, G., Rowe, M., & Miller, C. (1990). Frequent fallers: Leading groups to identify psychological factors. *Journal of Gerontological Nursing, 16*(4), 15-19.

Young, S. W., Abedzadeh, C. H., & White, M. W. (1989). A fall-prevention program for nursing homes. *Nursing Management, 20*(11), 80V-80AA, 80DD, 80FF.

Index

About the Author

Janice M. Morse is Professor of Nursing and Behavioral Science at the School of Nursing, The Pennsylvania State University. She has been studying patient falls since 1982 and extended this research to explore the effects of restraining patients and fall prevention measures. She has been involved in the development of a geriatric bed and a bed alarm. With doctorates in both nursing and anthropology, she has published extensively and is the editor of *Qualitative Health Research*.